Current Topics in Pathology
94

Springer
Berlin
Heidelberg
New York
Barcelona
Hong Kong
London
Milan
Paris
Singapore
Tokyo

R. Cerio (Ed.)

Dermatopathology

Contributors
J. E. Arrese, Y. Beguin, G. Burg, L. Cerroni, D. Innocenzi,
W. Kempf, H. Kerl, W. Mooi, P. Paquet, G. E. Piérard, S. Whittaker,
B. Zelger, B. G. Zelger

Springer

Dr. R. Cerio
Department of Morbid Anatomy and Histopathology
The Royal London Hospital
Whitechapel, London E1 1BB
Great Britain

With 74 Figures and 6 Tables

ISBN 3-540-67720-8 Springer-Verlag Berlin Heidelberg New York

Library of Congress Cataloging-in-Publication Data

Dermatopathology / Rino Cerio (ed.) ; contributors, D. Innocenzi ... [et al.].
p. ; cm. – (Current topics in pathology ; 94)
Includes bibliographical references and index.
ISBN 3540677208 (alk. paper)
1. Skin–Diseases. I. Cerio, Rino, 1956- II. Innocenzi, D. (Daniele) III. Current topics in pathology ; v. 94.
[DNLM: 1. Skin–pathology. 2. Skin Diseases–pathology. WR 105 D4353 2001]
RL96 .D477 2001
616.5′07–dc21
2001020001

Springer-Verlag Berlin Heidelberg New York
a member of BertelsmannSpringer Science+Business Media GmbH

http://www.springer.de

Production: PRO EDIT GmbH, Heidelberg
Cover design: Design & Production GmbH, Heidelberg
Typesetting: Fotosatz-Service Köhler GmbH, Würzburg

Printed on acid-free paper SPIN 10771336 24/3130/Di 5 4 3 2 1 0

Dedication

Dedicated to all practising and aspiring dermatopathologists

Contributors

J. E. Arrese	Centre Hospitalier Universitaire de Liège, Service de Dermapathologie, Institut de Pathologie, 1er étage, 4000 Liège, Belgium
Y. Beguin	Department of Haematology-Oncology, Centre Hospitalier Universitaire de Liège, 4000 Liège, Belgium
G. Burg	Dermatopathology, Universitätsspital Zurich, Gloriastr. 31, 8091 Zurich, Switzerland
L. Cerroni	Department of Dermatology, University of Graz, Auenbruggerplatz 8, 8036 Graz, Austria
D. Innocenzi	Università degli Studi la "Sapienza" Roma Italia, Viale del Policlinico, 155, 00161 Rome, Italy
W. Kempf	Department of Dermatology, University Hospital, 8091 Zurich, Switzerland
H. Kerl	Department of Dermatology and Venerology, University of Graz Medical School, Auenbrugger Platz 8, 8036 Graz, Austria
W. Mooi	Department of Pathology, The Netherlands Cancer Institute, Plesmanlaan 121, 1066 CX Amsterdam, The Netherlands

P. Paquet
Centre Hospitalier Universitaire de Liège,
Service de Dermatopathologie,
Institut de Pathologie, 1er étage,
4000 Liège, Belgium

G. E. Piérard
Centre Hospitalier Universitaire de Liège,
Service de Dermatopathologie,
Institut de Pathologie, 1er étage,
4000 Liège, Belgium

S. Whittaker
Consultant Dermatologist
Research Director,
St. John's Institute of Dermatology,
St. Thomas' Hospital,
Lambeth Palace Road,
London SE1 7EH, UK

B. Zelger
Department of Dermatology,
University of Innsbruck,
Anichstraße 35,
6020 Innsbruck, Austria

B. G. Zelger
Department of Pathology,
University of Innsbruck,
Müllerstraße 44, 6020 Innsbruck, Austria

Preface

Dermatology is one of the few remaining medical specialities that depends almost entirely on both physical examination and microscopic evaluation, i.e. clinicopathological correlation. However, over the last decade we have also witnessed a worldwide increase in recognition of dermatopathology as a sub-speciality, especially in Europe. There has been continued research in skin disease. Immunopathology and molecular pathology have provided further insight into pathogenesis, cell differentiation and re-classification of cutaneous infection, auto-immune disorders, skin cancers, fibrohistocytic lesions and lympho-proliferative disorders to mention but a few. The spread of human immunodeficiency virus (HIV) has put dermatopathological diagnosis in the front line, as affected individuals not only get unusual, sometimes unique and often multiple opportunistic infections, but also florid presentations of common dermatoses. This volume is directed at a wide audience including trainees in pathology and/or dermatology, the practising dermatopathologist, and both the generalist and researcher interested in aspects of skin pathology. It aims to be a guide to the interpretation of cutaneous biopsy sections especially in some of the more difficult areas such as Spitz-like melanocytic tumours, fibroproliferative tumours and B + T cell skin lymphoma. In addition, a chapter dedicated to the clinical pathological features of skin disorders in HIV and the pathological differential diagnosis of graft-versus-host disease compared with erythema multiforme is included. All authors have a national and international reputation and expertise in dermatopathology; some are trained in pathology, others in dermatology and most in both. Although each has personal opinions based on their education and training, all their contributions are aimed at helping those who work in dermatopathology to understand biological variations and avoid misdiagnosis.

The topics covered are obviously selected, and editing of the book has been rigorous. We expect this will serve our readers in several ways. Throughout the book a uniform style of presentation has been adopted. We have chosen to minimise historical and speculative information and where possible we avoided any duplication. The decision to use black and white photographs was made so that many more examples, than in previous editions, could be included within a limited budget. For histology, such photomicrographic interpretation can often be better appreciated.

It is the hope of the editor to not only update and encourage those trainees to become specialist dermatopathologists, but also to maintain the enthusiasm that a sound knowledge of dermatopathology can instil in all physicians who enjoy studying skin disease.

Consultant Dermatologist
and Senior Lecturer
in Dermatopathology

Dr. Rino Cerio,
BSc MBBS FRCP (Lon.)
FRCP (Edin.) DipRCPath

Contents

Skin Diseases Associated with HIV Infection

D. Innocenzi

1 Introduction

Although opportunistic infections are important causes of morbidity and mortality, noninfectious conditions frequently make substantial contributions to the disease course. Patients with HIV infection are at increased risk for neoplastic

Current Topics in Pathology
Volume 94; R. Cerio (Ed.)

diseases, both by decreased immunological response to abnormal cells and by increased susceptibility to infection by viruses. However, they do not have an increased incidence of the most common tumours affecting the general population, such us breast, colon, and prostate carcinoma.

The most common neoplastic conditions associated with HIV infection are Kaposi's sarcoma (KS), malignant lymphoma and cervical carcinoma. All of these malignant neoplastic diseases have been shown to have an association with a virus: KS with herpes hominis virus 8 (HHV-8), malignant lymphoma with Epstein-Barr virus (EBV), and cervical carcinoma with human papilloma virus (HPV). As of the end of 1998, and based on an extensive country-by-country review of HIV/AIDS data, 33.4 million adults are currently estimated to be alive and infected with HIV or to have AIDS. Of the total prevalent HIV infections, the majority remain concentrated in eastern, central and southern Africa, but the epidemic is evolving, with spread of infection from urban to rural areas, as well as to West and South Africa, India and Southeast Asia, and to a lesser extent with proportional shifts to heterosexual infections in North America, western Europe and Latin America. While the longer-term dimensions of the HIV epidemic at the global level cannot be forecast with confidence, the World Health Organisation (WHO) currently projects a cumulative total of close to 40 million HIV infections in men, women and children by the year 2000 [1].

Reports indicate that both death and incidence rates as well as the development of opportunistic infections have recently been drastically reduced. These reductions are due in part to improved prevention efforts but mainly to recent advances in the management of HIV infection, including the availability of new combination therapies such as highly active anti-retroviral therapy (HAART).

Diseases of the skin and mucous membranes were among the first recognised clinical manifestations of AIDS. Over the past decade it has become increasingly clear that cutaneous disorders are not only associated with terminal immunodeficiency but also occur throughout the course of HIV infection: more than 90% of patients develop skin or mucous membrane conditions at some time during their disease, and in many the skin is the first organ affected. Moreover, several skin diseases have proved to be sensitive and useful measures by which the progression of HIV can be monitored [2].

Two distinct populations of viruses are responsible for AIDS: HIV type 1 (HIV-1), the viral group responsible for AIDS in Central Africa and the rest of the world, and HIV type 2 (HIV-2), the viral group responsible for AIDS in West Africa. The main process of clinical disease progression is the functional abnormalities and quantitative depletion of CD4 T lymphocytes, which causes the profound immunosuppression characteristic of advanced HIV infection [3].

Evidence is accumulating to suggest the existence of two different subsets of T-helper (Th) $CD4^+$ cells: Th1 and Th2. Th1 cells preferentially develop during infections by intracellular bacteria and trigger phagocyte-mediated host defence, whereas Th2 cells, which predominate during helminthic infestations and in response to common environmental allergens, are responsible for phagocyte-independent host response. Th1 and Th2 cells exhibit not only different functional properties but probably also distinct surface markers. Clearly, polarised Th1 and Th2 responses not only play different roles in protection but can also promote different immunopathological reactions. A strong and persistent Th1 response seems to be involved in organ-specific autoimmunity, contact dermatitis and some chronic inflammatory disorders of unknown aetiology. In contrast, a polarised Th2 response favours a reduced protection against the majority of infectious agents (including HIV) and, in genetically predisposed hosts, is responsible for triggering allergic atopic disorders [4]. A predominant Th1 milieu occurs in the immunocompetent host. During the course of HIV infection there is a shift in cellular immunity from a Th1 immune response to a Th2 response, which may be modulated by IL-10. The Th1 response is associated with production of interferon-γ and IL-2, whereas the Th2 type of response is associated with IL-4, IL-5, IL-6 and IL-10. IL-4 and IL-5 induce IgE production and eosinophilia. Th2 cytokines may act as, or promote the activity of, associated angiogenic factors such as IL-1, IL-6 and TGF-β. These facts may explain the leading atopy, Kaposi's sarcoma, bacillary angiomatosis, and other pathologies developed in this milieu.

The natural history of HIV infection is divided into stages, as shown in Fig. 1. HIV is transmitted (a) across mucosal membranes by sexual contact, (b) through haematogenous exposure to virally contaminated blood or blood products and (c) from mother to foetus or neonate. In 50%–70% of patients with primary HIV infection an acute mononucleosis-like syndrome develops approximately 3–6 weeks after initial infection. Following primary infection, and with or without the appearance of HIV-specific immunity, most patients have a period of "clinical latency" that lasts for a median of 10 years. After this period we can observe either a persistent generalised lymphadenopathy (PGL), defined as enlarged lymph nodes involving at least two noncontiguous sites other than inguinal nodes, or the early symptomatic HIV infection with the AIDS-related complex (ARC), including conditions that are more common and more severe in the presence of HIV infection such as recurrent herpes zoster or oral hairy leucoplakia, but these symptoms are not AIDS-indicator conditions. As HIV infection progresses virtually every structure may be involved, and the progression to AIDS or death increases with a steeper CD4 decline [3–53]. The most important skin diseases associated with HIV infection will be discussed in this chapter.

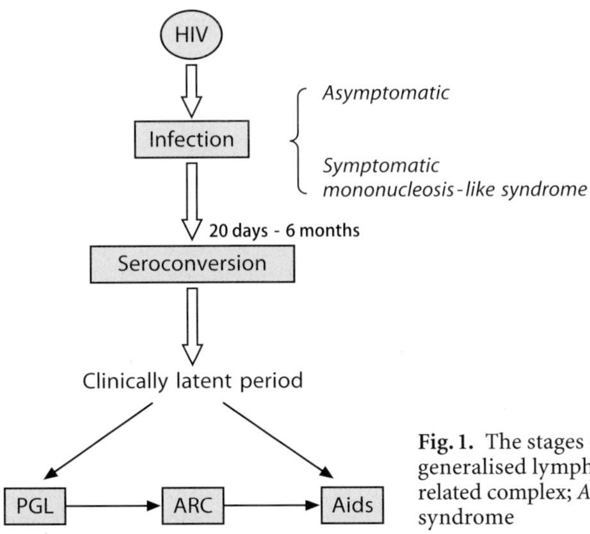

Fig. 1. The stages of HIV infection. *PGL*, Persistent generalised lymphadenopathy; *ARC*, AIDS-related complex; *AIDS*, acquired immunodeficiency syndrome

2 Viral Infections

2.1 Acute Exanthema in HIV Disease

The acute phase of HIV infection includes several manifestations, such as fever, sore throat, oral ulcers, lymphadenopathy, headache, myalgias, arthralgias, vomiting, diarrhoea and exanthema. Skin rash has been reported in 67%–72% of cases [5].The clinical picture is a nonpruritic, macular or maculopapular rash, without confluence and sometimes with desquamation [6–54]. The sites most commonly involved are the trunk, face, neck and upper extremities, but even the palms and the soles can be affected. In a few cases exanthema or small ulcers in the oral cavity have been noticed [7]. The intensity of the rash varies, and vesicles, sometimes progressing to small ulcers, can occur only in severe cases. The establishment of HIV antigen in serum, the isolation of HIV from cell-free plasma and from blood mononuclear cells in the absence of antibodies during the acute illness, and the disappearance of the antigen later on clearly indicate that in HIV infection, as in other generalised virus infections, there is a period of viremia preceding the antibody response. Many systemic viral diseases are accompanied by exanthema. It is known that this can either be due to a direct cytotoxic effect of the virus, as in varicella, or the result of a T-cell-mediated immunoreaction, as in rubella. Secondary syphilis is the main differential diagnosis of the HIV exanthema [6], such as pityriasis rosea, and other viral or drug-induced exanthemas. It must be emphasised that the histopathological features of HIV exanthema are not diagnostic for HIV infection, as the histology is the same as in many other virus infections [8].

Skin biopsy specimens show a lymphohistiocytic infiltrate around the vessels of the superficial plexus, and atypical mononuclear cells with a hyperchromatic nucleus have occasionally been reported [9]. Individual necrosis of keratinocytes and mild exocytosis have also been observed. The absence of epidermal changes other than a few lymphocytic cells in the lower part of the epithelium excludes pityriasis rosea.

2.2 Herpesvirus

Herpesvirus infections are among the most common viral opportunistic infections in persons with AIDS, accounting for approximately 16% of all clinically significant infections in these patients. The typical presentations of cutaneous herpes simplex virus (HSV) are well known and rarely cause diagnostic difficulty, although atypical forms of cutaneous HSV infection and atypical locations such as the buttocks and lower back have been reported in HIV-infected patients [10, 11]. HSV type 1 or type 2 cause typical herpetic vesicles on oral or genital mucosa, respectively. A survey of ulcers in those with AIDS [12] revealed that HSV was most frequently isolated once the CD4 T-cell count in the blood had dropped below 50×10^6/l. However, these lesions may progress to extensive ulceration, involving a greater skin surface area and deeper tissue. HSV may also initiate infection of some visceral organs that are only rarely involved in patients with normal immunity. Thus HSV may cause oesophagitis, pneumonitis or hepatitis in those with AIDS [12]. HSV encephalitis is not a significant problem in those with AIDS, probably because of their impaired ability to mount an inflammatory immune response [12]. HSV causing chronic mucocutaneous ulceration persisting for more than 1 month, or gastrointestinal, pulmonary and disseminated infection are included in the CDC definition of AIDS [10]. There is a correlation between the appearance of HSV-induced ulcerous lesions and CD4-cell levels below 50×10^6/l in HIV+ patients, and co-infection by HSV and HIV can adversely affect prognosis [13].

Herpes zoster occurs among HIV-infected individuals at an incidence about seven times greater than that in the general population [14]. The eruption often occurs as an early sign of compromised immune function, which makes it an important indicator of HIV infection among younger individuals.

The clinical presentation of herpes zoster in HIV-infected patients is often typical, with a dermal distribution, but some patients experience recurrent attacks [14]. Recently, atypical forms of varicella-zoster virus (VZV) infection in HIV-positive patients have been reported. Nodular, pox-like, hyperkeratotic or necrotic skin lesions in AIDS patients receiving prolonged treatment with acyclovir have been described [14]. However, disseminated zoster, defined as the occurrence of more than 25 extradermal lesions, has been infrequently reported in patients with HIV infection [15]. Disseminated infection has been associated with increased morbidity and mortality. The individual vesicles and pustules have been reported to be larger, with the development of extensive ulcerations and black eschara [15]. HSV and VZV develop identical histological patterns. The histopathology of the herpetic lesion reflects its age. Initially, changes are confined to the epidermis and consist of intraepidermal vesicles containing acantholytic and often multinucleated keratinocytes, frequently with eosinophilic intranuclear inclusions (Fig. 2). There is margination of chromatin with ballooning nuclear degeneration and pinkish intracytoplasmic and intranuclear inclusions known as Cowdry bodies [16]. A mixed infiltrate with lymphocytes, histiocytes, eosinophils, neutrophils and plasma cells may be observed in the dermis, with perineural and intraneural inflammation associated with degeneration of nerves [16]. Older lesions often show areas of necrosis and ulceration lacking these diagnostic features. Similar cyto-

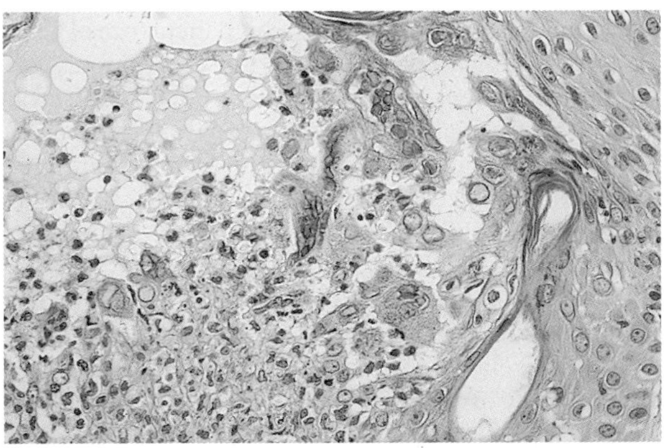

Fig. 2. Herpesvirus: intraepidermal vesicles containing acantholytic and multinucleated keratinocytes with eosinophilic intranuclear inclusions

pathic and acantholytic changes may also affect other epithelial structures, including those of eccrine glands.

The clinical diagnosis of HSV and VZV infection is confirmed by a positive Tzanck smear or biopsy specimen showing typical multinucleated giant cells.

The differential diagnosis of vesicular lesions in patients with AIDS includes herpes virus infection [17], cytomegalovirus infection, epidermolysis bullosa acquisita, dermatitis herpetiformis, bullous pemphigoid, enteroviral infection, and drug reaction [17]. It must be emphasised here, as above, that the histopathological features of HIV exanthema are not diagnostic for HIV infection as the histology is the same as in many other virus infections [8].

Verrucous skin lesions in HIV have been attributed to VZV, HSV and CMV. In their study of six patients with verrucous VZV infection and AIDS, Le Boit et al. [18] concluded that polymerase chain reaction studies should be a standard investigation to clarify the presence or absence of particular viruses, as they contend that HSV and CMV do not produce verrucous lesions. Chronic verrucous or eczematous VZV is seen almost exclusively in HIV disease, and it may occur after primary infection or reactivation. In chronic VZV painful, hyperkeratotic ulcerated plaques persist for months [18–55]. The distribution may be localised or disseminated.

The histopathological pattern of verrucous lesions shows a variable degree of verrucous epidermal hyperplasia, pseudocarcinomatous hyperplasia of adnexal epithelial structures, and massive hyperkeratosis. These striking findings correlate with the crusted, warty clinical appearance of the lesions.

The epithelial changes seen in these lesions somewhat resemble those seen in other chronic conditions such as deep fungal infections or blastomycosis-like pyoderma, and halogenodermia.

2.3 Cytomegalovirus

Cytomegalovirus (CMV) is an important source of morbidity and mortality in immunocompromised patients. Common CMV complications in patients with AIDS who have CD4 counts of less than 100 cells/mm^3 include retinitis, encephalitis, gastroenteritis, and pneumonia. There is some evidence that CMV accelerates the progression of HIV infection to clinical AIDS [20]. Despite the high incidence of CMV among HIV patients, cutaneous involvement is rare. The most commonly encountered skin lesions are chronic nonhealing ulcers. These are often localised in the perianal and perineal regions, and they usually represent spread from sites of contiguous CMV proctocolitis. Cytomegalovirus ulcers also occur on the oropharyngeal mucosa and other skin surfaces. Other reported presentations of cutaneous CMV infection include verrucous plaques, vesiculobullous eruptions, purpuric maculopapular eruptions, leucocytoclastic vasculitis, and cutaneous thrombosis [56].

CMV typically induces cell enlargement and produces large basophilic nuclear inclusions with a broad surrounding halo or eosinophilic cytoplasmic inclusions, or both. The altered cells are most often endothelial cells and fibroblasts; however, sweat gland and epidermal involvement in patients with HIV disease have been reported [21].

2.4 Oral Hairy Leucoplakia

Oral hairy leucoplakia (OHL), Burkitt's lymphoma and large-cell lymphoma represent Epstein-Barr (EB) virus diseases that can be observed in HIV-infected patients. OHL is a benign hyperplasia of the oral mucosa, first reported by Greesporen et al. in a homosexual man, that has subsequently been shown to occur in HIV-negative patients who are immunosuppressed. Recently, OHL has also been reported in nonimmunosuppressed patients. OHL is a frequent finding in patients with HIV, indicates advanced immunosuppression and, in patients with more than 300/µl $CD4^+$ lymphocytes, is associated with a poor prognosis [22].

Clinically, it is characterised by bilateral, elevated, white patches on the lateral surface of the tongue that may extend to the dorsal or ventral surfaces (Fig. 3). Furthermore, same cases have been described on the cheek mucosa, soft palate, pharynx and oesophagus.

Histopathologically, there is hyperkeratosis and acanthosis of the epithelium with minimal inflammatory infiltrate in the corium (Fig. 4). Clusters of keratino-

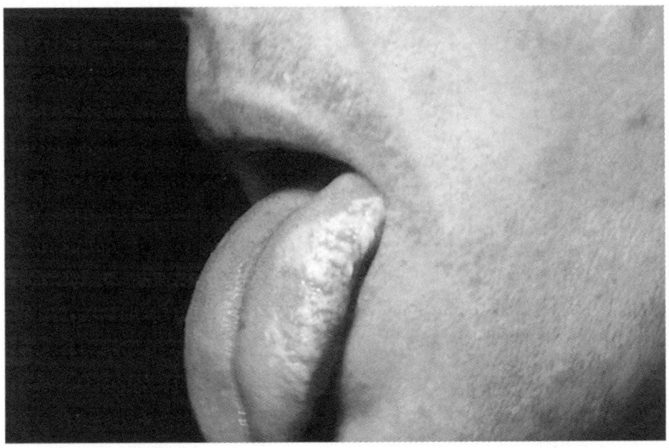

Fig. 3. Oral hairy leucoplakia: white patches on the lateral surface of the tongue

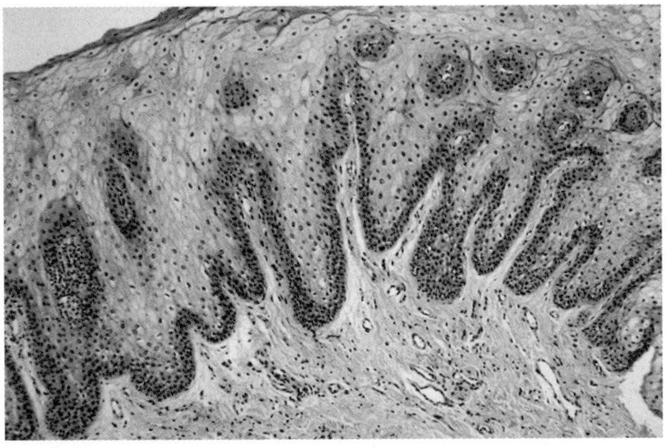

Fig. 4. Oral hairy leucoplakia: hyperkeratosis and acanthosis of the epithelium with minimal inflammatory infiltrate in the dermis

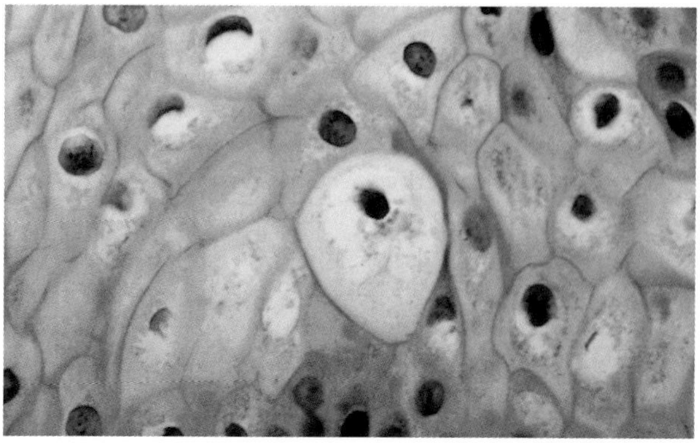

Fig. 5. Oral hairy leucoplakia: keratinocytes in ballooning degeneration

cytes show ballooning degeneration (Fig. 5) and some beaded nuclei or ground-glass intranuclear inclusions may be observed [23]. EBV replicating vegetatively in histological or cytological specimens is required for definitive diagnosis. There is not a specific histopathological pattern of OHL because fungus infection, or biting or other traumatic events could cause the same lesions [24]. The differential diagnosis includes other ballooning degenerative lesions of the mouth, including chronic maceration and white sponge nevus.

2.5 Human Papillomavirus Infection

The incidence of human papilloma virus (HPV) skin diseases has been shown to be increased in immunodeficient individuals. Patients who have undergone transplantation and individuals with compromised immune systems have demonstrated an increased risk of developing HPV infections. Many studies have shown a marked increase in concomitant HPV infection in the cervical, perianal, anal, and penile regions in HIV-seropositive subjects as compared with individuals who have normal immune systems [25].

HPV is a double-stranded circular DNA virus identified as the causative agent of condyloma acuminatum, common verrucae and other epithelial proliferative lesions. The HPVs are broadly grouped into mucosal and cutaneous types, based on the clinical location of infection. Some overlap does exist, and certain HPV subtypes may be present at both sites. The HPV lesions usually manifest as benign epithelial appendages that may appear as acuminatous, papular, or flat lesions [25]. At least 82 different HPV types have been identified, based on the DNA sequence diversity, and many remain yet uncharacterised [26]. Different HPV phenotypes are associated with different diseases; HPVs associated with genital disease are divided into low-risk, intermediate-risk and high-risk viruses, according to their prevalence in cancers [27].

Types 1, 2, and 4 cause common warts and plantar warts. The basic morphology of common warts occurring in HIV disease is similar to that in the immunocompetent population. These lesions appear as circumscribed, rough, hard, hyperkeratotic verrucous papules or nodules, often with visible thrombosed capillaries and an irregular scaly surface, most commonly involving the hands, fingers and knees. On mucous membranes, warts often display less hyperkeratosis, and may then be pedunculated. In some cases, warts coalesce into plaques or cauliflower-like masses. The histological features of verruca vulgaris are papillomatosis, marked hyperkeratosis, acanthosis and parakeratosis. Elongated rete ridges at the edge of the lesion exhibit an inward bowing at the base, referred to as arborisation. Three histopathological features used to distinguish the common warts from other papillomas include the presence of koilocytes, vertical columns of parakeratosis, and foci of clumped keratohyaline granules [28]. The dermal changes in verruca vulgaris tend to be minimal. About 8% are inflamed and demonstrate a lichenoid infiltrate [28]. Palmoplantar or myrmecial warts in HIV-positive patients may appear as hard nodules or thick endophytic plaques larger and more numerous than those found in HIV-negative individuals, typically on the palms and/or soles [29]. Histopathologically, they show vacuolated cells in the epidermis with eosinophilic granules that coalesce to form large, irregularly shaped, homogeneous inclusion bodies [57, 58]. Small intranuclear eosinophilic inclusion bodies may be noted within cells of the upper stratum malpighii. Sometimes parakeratosis may be observed [28].

Types 5 and 8 are associated with epidermodysplasia verruciformis (EDV), a rare skin disorder in which HPV infection and a cell-mediated immunodeficiency lead to the development of squamous cell skin cancers [30]. Clinically, lesions of EDV are polymorphic, with a verruca plana-like appearance, localised to the dorsum of the hands and extremities, or a pityriasis versicolor-like aspect found on the trunk, pubic area, neck and face [28]. Lesions that remain unresponsive to aggressive therapy should be sampled and evaluated for intraepithelial dysplasia [31]. The flat warts of EDV resemble other examples of verruca plana architecturally but have a distinctive cytopathic difference. Rather than the prominent perinuclear halos seen in common verruca plana, the keratinocytes of the middle and upper spinous layer have abundant, finely granular, basophilic cytoplasm, the result of a profusion of ribosomes in infected cells [32].

Histologically, these lesions are characterised by swollen, pale, slightly basophilic keratinocytes containing keratohyaline granules of variable size and shape clustered in the granular and spinous layer of the epidermis [28]. The stratum corneum is loose, with a basket-weave appearance.

Types 6 and 11 are associated primarily with condylomata acuminata of the anogenital region and laryngeal papilloma, and frank neoplastic changes are uncommon when only these types are present. Types 16 and 18 are generally believed to confer a high risk of invasive anogenital cancer, whereas types 31, 33 and 35 are associated with an intermediate risk of progression to malignancy. These so-called oncogenic HPV genotypes (HPV 16, 18 and 31) have been detected in 80%–90% of cervical intraepithelial neoplasia (CIN) grade 3 lesions and invasive cervical cancers [59]. Studies from the era prior to the introduction of highly active antiretroviral therapy (HAART) have shown that the prevalence of anal infection with HPV and anal squamous intraepithelial lesions (ASIL) were high among HIV-positive homosexual men, and to a lesser extent among HIV-negative homosexual men. The data also show that the incidence of high-grade ASIL (HSIL), the putative invasive cancer precursor lesion, was high in these groups. Early data suggest that at least 75% of those with HSIL lesions do not regress while receiving HAART.

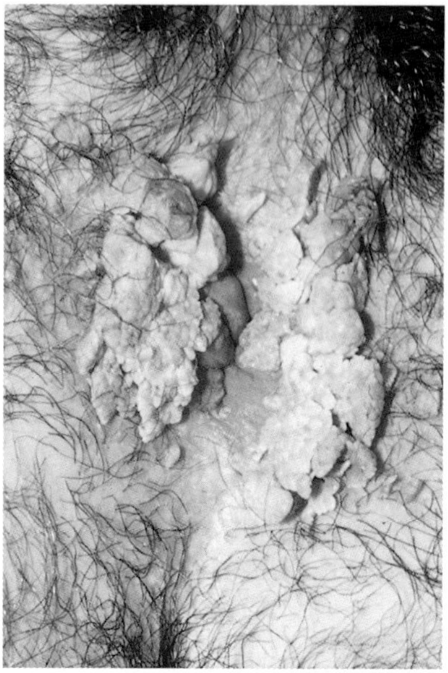

Fig. 6. Condyloma acuminatum: multiple lesions of the vulva

Given that progression of HSIL to invasive cancer may require several years, lengthened survival associated with HAART may paradoxically lead to an increased risk of anal cancer. Probably, the normal immune mechanism prevents latent anal HPV infection from causing neoplasia. When this mechanism is impaired as a consequence of HIV infection, HPV can become active in promoting the development of premalignant epithelial lesions. Clinically, condylomata acuminata generally present as single or multiple papules or nodules most commonly seen on the penis, vulva, vagina, cervix, perineum and anal region (Fig. 6) [33]. These lesions may progress to large pedunculated, exophytic, cauliflower-like masses typically seen on most non-hair-bearing skin of the perineum [28].

Histologically, the epidermis in condyloma acuminatum appears undulating and moderately acanthotic with mild hyperkeratosis (Fig. 7), a prominent granular

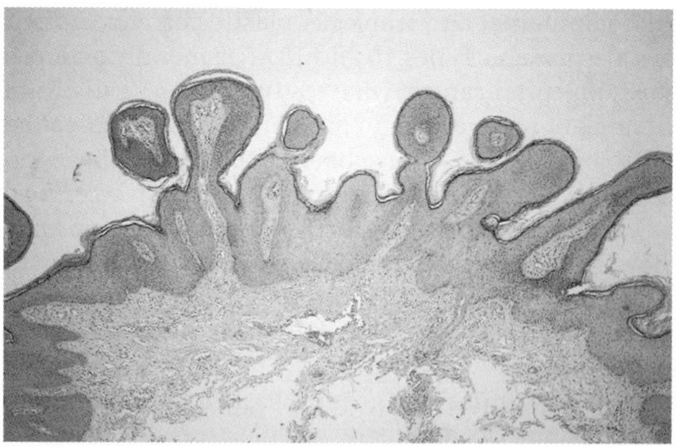

Fig. 7. Condyloma acuminatum: moderate acanthosis with mild hyperkeratosis of the epidermis, which appears undulating

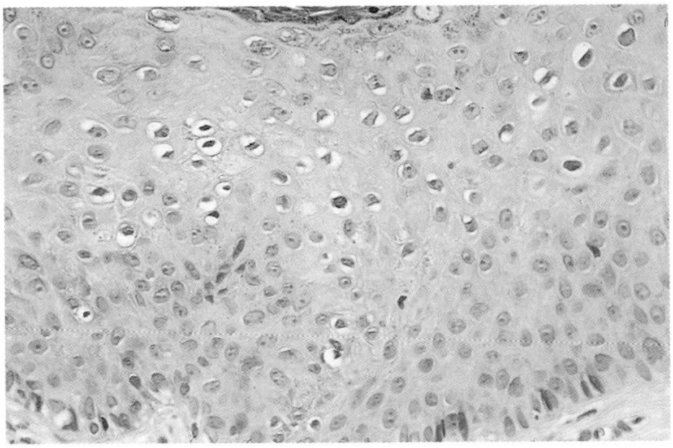

Fig. 8. Condyloma acuminatum: koilocytes in the malpighian layer

layer with coarse keratohyaline granules and koilocytes (Fig. 8). These cells tend to aggregate in the superficial malpighian and granular layer. Lesions treated with podophyllin exhibit numerous necrotic keratinocytes and a marked increase in the number of mitotic figures arrested in metaphase in the lower half of the epidermis. This histopathological presentation can be confused with squamous cell carcinoma in situ or with bowenoid papulosis.

Bowenoid papulosis (BP) occurs predominantly in young, sexually active adults, 20–35 years old [60]. BP presents with multiple wart-like brown-red papules an average of 7 mm in diameter in the anogenital region that histologically resemble in situ squamous cell carcinoma [60]. Sometimes the papules become confluent and coalesce. The lesion may be mistaken for lichen planus, psoriasis, seborrhoeic keratosis or condyloma acuminatum [61]. A viral aetiology has been well documented in BP; HPV 16 has been detected in the majority of cases. HPVs 18, 31, 32, 34, 35, 39, 42, 48 and 51 through 54 are also occasionally detected.

BP is characterised by psoriasiform hyperplasia and hyperkeratosis of the epidermis. Keratinocytes appear crowded and display enlarged hyperchromatic and pleomorphic nuclei. Increased numbers of mitotic figures, some atypical, are seen at all epidermal levels. This aspect seems to be similar to squamous cell carcinoma findings [34].

The differential diagnosis of BP is wide and includes lichen planus, psoriasis, seborrhoeic keratosis, pyogenic granuloma and condyloma acuminatum.

2.6 Molluscum Contagiosum

Molluscum contagiosum (MC) is a benign self-limited viral infection which, although usually dismissed as a banal disease, should alert dermatologists and venereologists because of the possibility of HIV infection. In fact, the lesions of MC develop in at least 20% of patients with AIDS. The aetiological agent is a DNA virus, a member of the pox family of viruses of which there are two strains, MCV1 and MCV2.

Although the pathogenesis of MC is poorly understood, there is evidence that the host cellular immunoresponse is crucial to the control of this viral infection. A

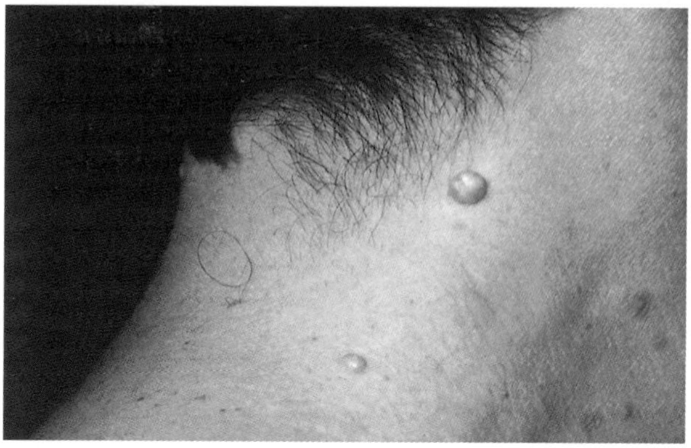

Fig. 9. Molluscum contagiosum: giant lesion on the neck

correlation between the low CD4+ count and the extent of the disease has been observed. MC clinically appears as dome-shaped umbilicated multiple translucid papulonodular lesions which can be observed on different areas of the body, mainly on the genitalia and face (Fig. 9). In the immunocompetent host, lesions often undergo spontaneous resolution. In immunocompromised patients the disease runs a chronic relapsing course, and atypical lesions with either multiple small [35] papules or giant nodular tumours can be observed.

Histologically, a central umbilication with epidermal hyperplasia is evident at scanning (Fig. 10). The superficial keratinocytes contain a very large eosinophilic intracytoplasmic inclusion which compresses the nucleus against the cell membrane (Fig. 11). The surrounding dermis usually shows little or no inflammatory reaction, except in instances in which the lesion of MC ruptures and discharges molluscum bodies and horny material into the dermis [36].

A differential diagnosis to cryptococcosis, cutaneous pneumocystosis and other infection diseases appearing similar to CM clinically must be made, and a skin biopsy is often necessary to exclude other diseases. Solitary lesions can clinically mimic pyogenic granuloma, keratoacanthoma or epithelioma and, in exceptional cases, sebaceous naevus, eczema or giant condyloma acuminatum.

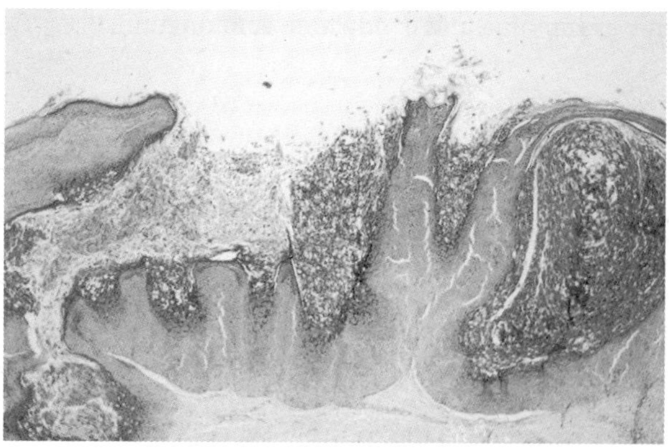

Fig. 10. Molluscum contagiosum: a central umbilication with epidermal hyperplasia is evident at scanning magnification

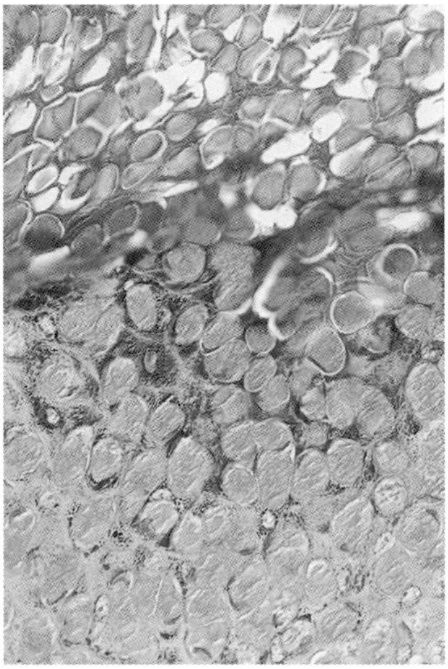

Fig. 11. Molluscum contagiosum: eosinophilic intracytoplasmic inclusions which compress the nucleus against the cell membrane

3 Bacterial Infections

3.1 Folliculitis, Furunculosis, Impetigo, Ecthyma

Although HIV-infected individuals are susceptible to multiple bacterial pathogens, *Staphylococcus aureus* is the most commonly encountered bacterial pathogen in HIV disease. Studies have documented the *S. aureus* nasal carriage rate in HIV-infected patients to be twice that of control groups [37]. It is known that in AIDS the migration and chemotactic response of neutrophils is markedly selective [38]. In fact delayed migration of neutrophils enhances the ability of the bacteria to produce disease [38]. Primary cutaneous infections include impetigo, folliculitis, furunculosis and ecthyma [31]. Atypical presentations are common and include plaque-like folliculitis, *Candida*-like intertrigo, and molluscum-like dermatoses [31]. In these immunocompromised hosts, recurrence is very common. Classic staphylococcal toxin syndromes have also been reported in HIV infection [39]. Additionally, a prolonged, recalcitrant desquamative erythroderma associated with staphylococcal toxins has been observed in AIDS patients [40]. Secondary infections and superinfections due to *S. aureus* frequently develop in HIV-infected patients with underlying dermatoses. Staphylococcal bacteraemia may complicate cutaneous staphylococcal infections, and fatal staphylococcal sepsis may occur. Histologically, folliculitis shows a dense infiltrate of mononuclear cells, surrounded and involved follicular structures with focal areas of suppurative folliculitis, and a few hair shaft fragments surrounded by histiocytes and giant cells [38]. Impetigo presents subcorneal pustules often with numerous gram-positive bacteria seen within the stratum corneum.

3.2 Bacillary Angiomatosis

Bacillary angiomatosis (BA), predominantly reported in the American literature, is a rare cutaneous disorder usually affecting patients with HIV infection and often misdiagnosed as a vascular tumour. In 1983, Stoler et al. [41] reported a patient with AIDS who had an atypical subcutaneous infection that was recognised retrospectively to be the first recorded case of BA.

The causal agents are two closely related species of a slow-growing, gram-negative bacilli, named *Rochalimaea quintana* and *Rochalimaea henselae* [42]. The pathogenesis is not completely known, but it has been postulated that a vasoproliferative factor either is produced by the bacterium itself or is induced to be formed by the host as a consequence of bacterial infection.

BA characteristically develops rapidly as a cutaneous vascular disorder. Clinically, lesions present as either solitary, scattered or widespread, superficial and deep angiomatous papules or nodules, sometimes leaking serosanguineous fluid. They often have a collarette of peripheral scale, closely resembling a pyogenic granuloma (Fig. 12).

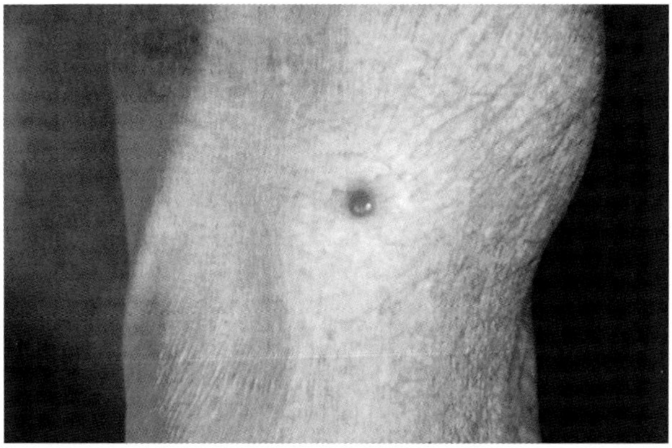

Fig. 12. Bacillary angiomatosis: papulonodular vascular lesion of the arm

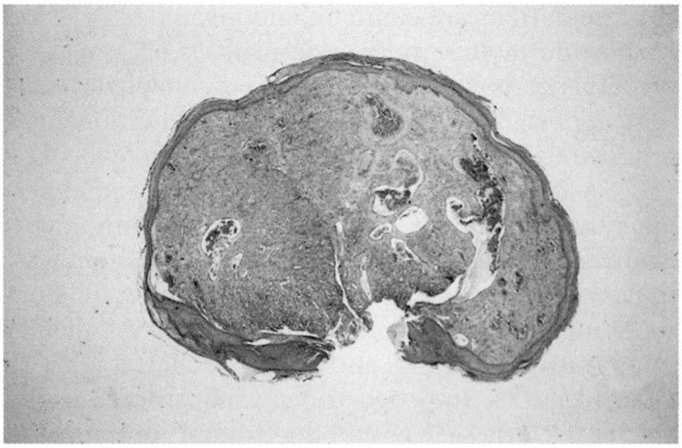

Fig. 13. Bacillary angiomatosis: well-circumscribed lobular capillary proliferation

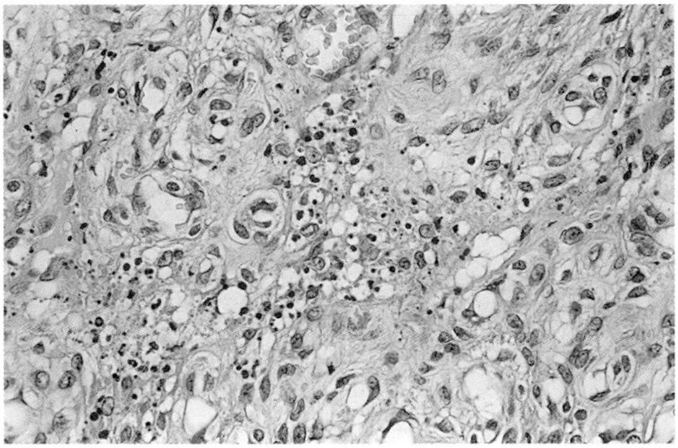

Fig. 14. Bacillary angiomatosis: blood vessels lined by large endothelial cells in an oedematous stroma containing scattered polymorphonuclear leucocytes and neutrophil debris

The clinical differential diagnosis also includes haemangioma, Kaposi's sarcoma and various subcutaneous tumours. BA can affect any cutaneous or mucous membrane. Systemic involvement includes organs such as the liver, spleen, bone and gastrointestinal tract. In very rare circumstances, it can present as soft tissue tumours without overlying skin signs. Systemic symptoms of weight loss, fever, chills and malaise may occur. Central nervous system manifestations, such as personality changes, have also been described.

The microscopic architectural features of BA are those of a well-circumscribed lobular capillary proliferation of blood vessels lined by large (epithelioid) endothelial cells that may show cytological atypia and mitotic activity, in an oedematous stroma containing scattered polymorphonuclear leucocytes and neutrophil debris (Fig. 13). Routine H&E sections sometimes show a granular basophilic material frequently adjacent to the vascular channels (Fig. 14). These represent numerous bacilli and are not always demonstrable by the Warthin-Starry stain (Fig. 15).

Ultrastructural examination reveals clusters of bacilli that usually lie between collagen bundles and contain an electron-dense centre surrounded by a trilaminar

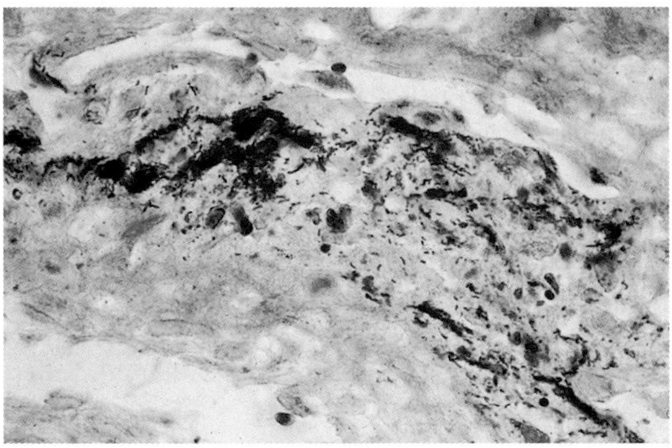

Fig. 15. Bacillary angiomatosis: numerous bacilli demonstrated by the Warthin-Starry stain

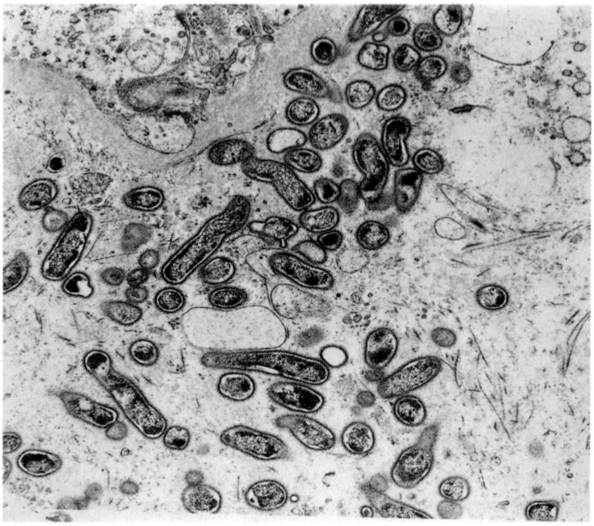

Fig. 16. Bacillary angiomatosis: clusters of bacilli demonstrated with electron microscopy

cell wall (Fig. 16). Histologically, it may resemble several other vascular tumours such as pyogenic granuloma, Kaposi's sarcoma, epithelioid haemangioma and, in some cases, angiosarcoma [43].

3.3 Mycobacteriosis

HIV infection has altered the epidemiology of mycobacterial infection. Recently, the incidence of mycobacteriosis has increased dramatically in all countries as a result of the HIV epidemic [44]. Patients with AIDS may assume a number of different clinical variants of mycobacterial skin lesions as oral ulcers, palmar and plantar hyperkeratosis, sporotricotic nodules, suppurative lymphadenitis, atopic dermatitis-like eruption, disseminated papules, pustules, vesicles and ulcers, and localised cutaneous abscesses. There are three mechanisms for the development of clinical tuberculosis in people with AIDS: reactivation of latent clinical tuberculosis, progression from recent infection and re-infection. A renewed interest in mycobacterial infections has also been kindled by the occurrence of *Mycobacterium avium* infections in patients with AIDS. Especially observed are disseminated infections when the $CD4^+$ cell count is low while TB occurs when $CD4^+$ counts are higher, between 250 and 500/nl. *Mycobacterium marinum* may cause classic swimming pool granulomata in patients with HIV disease [45]. Numerous other *Mycobacteria* may induce skin infections in HIV-infected patients Histologically, different features are observed, from non-caseating granuloma, to caseating granuloma, to an absence of granuloma. In general, the cellular response is characterised by epithelioid macrophages, Langhans giant cells and caseous necrosis, with perivascular lymphocytes in the surrounding tissue (tuberculous granuloma). Tubercle bacilli can be present, particularly in the areas of necrosis.

3.4 Syphilis

There is a strong epidemiological association between historical and serological evidence of past infection with *Treponema pallidum* (or any genital ulcer disease) and the risk of HIV infection [46]. The similarities between syphilis and AIDS are striking in many respects. Both diseases are sexually transmitted. In the industrialised world, both heterosexual and homosexual transmission (between male homosexual partners) is common, as is sexual transmission among needle-sharing, intravenous drug users and their partners [47]. In the developing world, heterosexual transmission is much more common, and the use of unscreened blood products may be important in both HIV and syphilis transmission. In contrast to the classic description of secondary syphilis [48], cutaneous secondary syphilis in HIV-infected patients is often associated with unusual clinical features. Oral erosions, nodules, papules, vesicles, hyperkeratotic plaques, and papulosquamous and maculopapular eruptions have all been described. Although the unusual manifestations of syphilis may be encountered in immunocompetent hosts, the likelihood of such is greater in HIV-infected patients with altered immunity, especially when the CD4 cell number drops below 150 cells/ml^3 [48].

Congenital infection is common to both illnesses and may occur in as many as one third of infants born to HIV-infected mothers [47]. Unlike infants with syphilis, most congenitally infected HIV-positive infants will die in the first few years of life. In adults, both diseases are characterised by long periods of latency following a symptomatic primary infection. The majority of syphilitics remain in latency with no long-term sequelae, whereas most patients with HIV infection will became clinically immunosuppressed with time. Neither organism is routinely culturable and the diagnosis of both diseases is based on clinical serological data [47]. In HIV-1-positive individuals, atypical and aggressive clinical manifestations of syphilis have been described. Syphilis skin manifestations similar to those in early reports of "malignant" syphilis may been seen [49]. Several reports have described atypical skin lesions of syphilis in HIV-positive individuals. In HIV-seropositive individuals, syphilis involving the eye has received special notice by several ophthalmologists. These ocular manifestations often are difficult to discern from cytomegalovirus- or HIV-induced eye diseases. The occurrence of accelerated progression to neurosyphilis with more aggressive characteristics has been reported [49]; this was explained by a potentiating effect of HIV on syphilitic infection. Invasion of the central nervous system by *T. pallidum* can already occur in the early stage of syphilis. A problem is whether neurological impairment is due to HIV infection, syphilis, or another entity. Although early syphilis in HIV-infected individuals usually is accompanied by reactive serological treponemal test results, false-negative results in HIV-positive patients have been reported [49]. Dark-field examination and special stains to detect treponemes in patients (silver staining, direct fluorescent antibody staining) remain highly important in the diagnosis of syphilis.

When skin biopsy specimens of lesions caused by *T. pallidum* are examined histologically, a variety of histopathological patterns may be seen. All reported cases of HIV-associated secondary syphilis in which the histopathological features were described demonstrated superficial and deep inflammatory cell infiltrates of lymphocytes, histiocytes, and plasma cells similar to those seen in immunocompetent counterparts. The epidermis is frequently involved, with exocytosis, spongiosis, parakeratosis and acanthosis being the most frequent changes. In late secondary lesions the infiltrate may become granulomatous [48].

In controversial cases the diagnosis can be confirmed by immunoperoxidase techniques using rabbit polyclonal or mouse monoclonal antibodies to *T. pallidum*. There does not appear to be a correlation between the nature and intensity of the inflammatory infiltrate, the number of treponemes, the syphilis serological titre, and the CD4 cell count in those cases in which all these data were available. Although histological manifestation may be protean, a superficial and deep lymphohistiocytic infiltrate with plasma cells and epidermal hyperplasia is the most common pattern of inflammation observed. Special stains for *T. pallidum* in tissue may aid in making an accurate diagnosis, especially in patients with false-negative results on serological tests for syphilis [48].

4 Parasitic and Protozoan Infections

4.1 Scabies

Scabies is a frequent cutaneous disease in HIV patients; it may be more severe and extensive than in immunocompetent hosts and can show involvement of atypical areas. Unusual clinical forms of scabies in HIV/AIDS are reported: hyperkeratosis plaques on the soles, trunk and extremities, bullous pemphigoid-like eruption [52]. Norwegian or crusted scabies can take atypical forms such as crusting with pruritus or a pruritic papular dermatitis and may resemble Darier's disease or psoriasis. HIV-infected patients with classic scabies often harbour an increased number of mites and are more infectious than immunocompetent hosts.

Scabies is an infection with the mite *Sarcoptes scabiei*, which excavates a burrow in the stratum corneum, where it lays numerous eggs that hatch in about 1 week. It is transmitted through prolonged contact or by clothing, clotheslines and towels. It is important to document infestation by scraping or skin biopsy, although scrapings obtained in the early stages of infestation may fail to reveal the mite. Because of the occurrence of nosocomial outbreaks of scabies, microscopic examination of skin scrapings in all AIDS patients with a generalised dermatitis has been recommended. Microscopic identification of mites, eggs and/or faeces confirms the diagnosis.

Histological examination usually shows a burrow located in the horny layer. Only the extreme blind end of the burrow, where the female mite is situated, extends into the stratum malphigii [50]. Spongiosis is present in the stratum malpighii near the mite to such an extent that formation of the vesicle is often the result. The dermal infiltrate in sections containing mites shows varying numbers of eosinophils. Papular-nodular lesions not containing mites show a nonspecific picture in which eosinophils generally are absent.

In Norwegian scabies innumerable mites are visible in the horny layer with a hyperplastic epidermis. In the superficial and mid dermis a perivascular and interstitial infiltrate of lymphocytes is observed. In post-scabies dermatitis a dense mixed inflammatory infiltrate with numerous eosinophils in nodular configuration resembling a pseudolymphoma may be seen. In nodular scabies mites are nearly absent [51].

4.2 *Pneumocystis carinii*

Cutaneous pneumocystosis in HIV-infected patients is quite rare and has a highly variable morphological presentation [62]. Although general pathologists are familiar with the appearance of the infected lung tissue, dermatopathologists may be unaware of either its appearance or its rare occurrence outside the lungs. Several patients have been reported as having disseminated *Pneumocystis* infection that involved the middle ear, presenting as a polyp protruding from the external auditory canal [56]. Widespread violaceous papules and nodules mimicking Kaposi's sarcoma have been described [63]. Blue maculae and molluscum-like papules have also been observed [64, 65]. Microemboli containing *P. carinii* have been reported in a patient with disseminated pneumocystosis and acral gangrene. The subepithelial connective tissue of cutaneous pneumocystosis has the same pink, frothy appearance on routinely stained sections as that seen in alveolar spaces on lung biopsy. On Gomori's methenamide silver stain or immunoperoxidase staining with anti-*Pneumocystis* antibody, the characteristic cysts and trophozoites can be demonstrated.

5 Systemic Fungal Infections

Cutaneous disease attributable to fungi are among the most common infections seen in HIV-positive patients, and their management poses special challenges [66]. Although many of these infections are not life threatening, they are the source of considerable morbidity. Moreover, they may predispose patients to other more serious types of infections that may be life threatening. For example, abnormalities in the skin produced by superficial fungal infections may provide the port of entry for streptococci, staphylococci, or gram-negative organisms [66]. A specific report of the most important fungal infection in HIV patients is provided below.

5.1 Candidiasis

In known HIV-infected individuals oral candidiasis is a reliable predictor of immune deterioration [67, 68]. Candidiasis is the most common oral opportunistic infection seen in patients with HIV infection and occurs in more than 90% of HIV-positive patients at some point during their disease [69]. There are four major clinical types of oral candidiasis, and all can be associated with HIV infection:

- Acute pseudomembranous (thrush)
- Erythematous (atrophic)
- Angular cheilitis
- Hyperplastic candidiasis

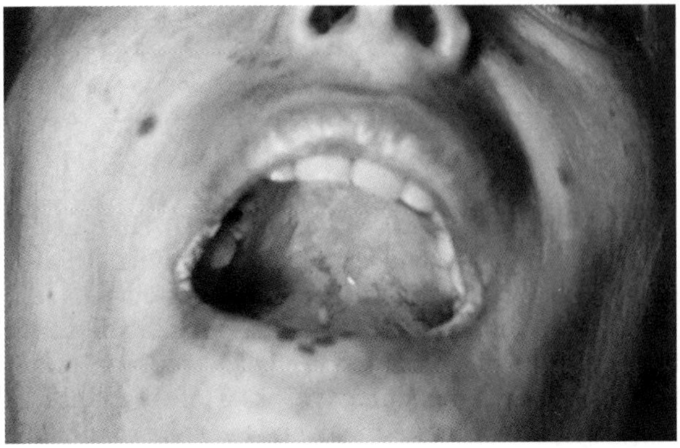

Fig. 17. Hyperplastic candidiasis: white plaque on the buccal mucosa with angular cheilitis

The *acute pseudomembranous form* is characterised by adherent white plaques localised to a discrete area of oral mucosa or, in immunocompromised patients, by yellowish or bluish-white plaques that cover large portions of the mouth. Diagnosis is made by demonstration of yeast or mycelia in smears that can be detected by potassium hydroxide, periodic acid-Schiff test, or Gram's stain.

The *erythematous form* presents as red macular lesions, most frequently involving the palate and dorsal surface of the tongue, where erythema often is accompanied by atrophy of the lingual papillae. This form of the disease is common and is as good a predictor of HIV infection as the pseudomembranous type [70].

Angular cheilitis presents as erythema and cracking of the commissures of the lips.

Hyperplastic candidiasis occurs when the fungus invades the deeper layer of the epithelium, resulting in acanthosis, parakeratosis and pseudoepitheliomatous hyperplasia. The lesions appear as firm white plaques on the buccal and labial mucosa or tongue that cannot be scraped off (Fig. 17). A biopsy stained with periodic acid-Schiff will show hyphae invading the epithelium (Fig. 18).

Intertriginous infection can involve the groin, axillary vault, or inframammary areas. A hallmark of *Candida* intertrigo is the presence of satellite pustules. *Candida* paronychia is also common [71].

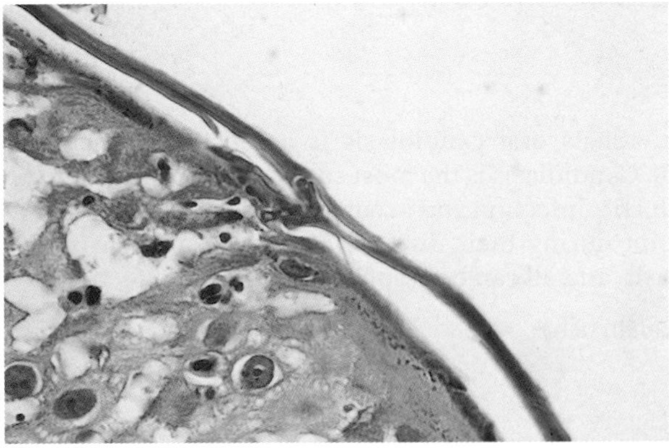

Fig. 18. Candidiasis: hyphae in the epithelium

5.2 Histoplasmosis

Disseminated histoplasmosis, caused by *Histoplasma capsulatum*, is not unusual in AIDS patients. Clinically, mucocutaneous lesions are highly variable in morphology and occur in about 10% of AIDS patients with disseminated histoplasmosis [72]. Papular and papulonecrotic lesions involving the face, trunk, and upper extremities are most common. Other morphologies include pustules, abscesses, nodules, umbilicated papules, ulcers and erythematous scaly plaques. Maculopapular exanthema, vegetative lesions, oral ulcers, and perianal ulcers are also observed [73]. Histological features range from tuberculoid granulomas with areas of necrosis, to accumulation of macrophages containing abundant organisms with a surrounding clear halo, to *Histoplasma* free in the dermis with little associated inflammation. Epidermal ulceration may be present, and transepidermal elimination has been described [74].

5.3 Sporotrichosis

Disseminated *Sporotrichosis schenchii* infection, showing granulomatous inflammation with giant cells containing budding yeast within the dermis, has also been described as occurring in HIV-infected patients [74].

5.4 Cryptococcosis

Cryptococcosis affects 5%–10% of HIV-infected individuals [75], and it is the fourth leading cause of opportunistic infection among this population [76]. It is caused by *Cryptococcus neoformans*.

Primary cryptococcosis is acquired by inhalation of the yeasts, resulting in a pulmonary infection that is often asymptomatic. Most often, disseminated cryptococcosis occurs by haematogenous spread from the lungs and may involve the meninges, brain, skin, bone and kidney.

Cryptococcal meningitis occurs in 80%–90% of patients who have both cryptococcosis and HIV disease. Approximately 10% of all immunocompromised patients with disseminated cryptococcosis will manifest cutaneous lesions [56], and the skin represents the most common site of extraneural disease. The cutaneous manifestations most frequently described are 0.2- to 1.0-cm umbilicated or crusted papules on the face or neck. Biopsies of the lesions show encapsulated organisms with minimal inflammatory response. Histopathologically, numerous encapsulated organisms are seen, located in a pale dermis with minimal inflammation.

5.5 Superficial Dermatophytosis

The incidence of dermatophytosis of the glabrous skin in HIV-positive patients is about 40% [66]. Tinea pedis is most frequent and is similar in appearance to the disease in non-HIV-infected persons. Tinea corporis, cruris and faciei, simulating seborrhoeic dermatitis, are also relatively common and are caused in most instances by the same organisms that cause disease in non-HIV-infected patients. Although superficial mycoses are easily treated, they frequently recur in this immunosuppressed population. Thus the major problem is to prevent recurrences. Generalised chronic dermatophytosis has been reported to occur in patients with a CD4 T cell count of less than 200 cells/mm^3 [77].

6 Noninfectious Skin Disorders

6.1 Seborrhoeic Dermatitis

Seborrhoeic dermatitis (SD) is the most common cutaneous disease observed in AIDS patients. It is more frequent in persons infected with the human immunodeficiency virus (20%–83%) than in HIV-negative persons (1%–3%) [78]. It is an inflammatory, erythematous and scaling eruption that occurs over the scalp, face, interscapular and presternal areas.

Clinically, the lesions of SD of AIDs are often indistinguishable from those of ordinary seborrhoeic dermatitis (Fig. 19). Differences include the greater severity of the former, its occurrence in a younger population, and the involvement of areas not typically involved in seborrhoeic dermatitis, such as the trunk and the extremities. The role of *Pityrosporum ovale* in the inflammatory process has been suggested in several studies: in fact, double-blind trials with antifungal drugs have reported a decrease of disease intensity [79]. The strong skin colonisation with

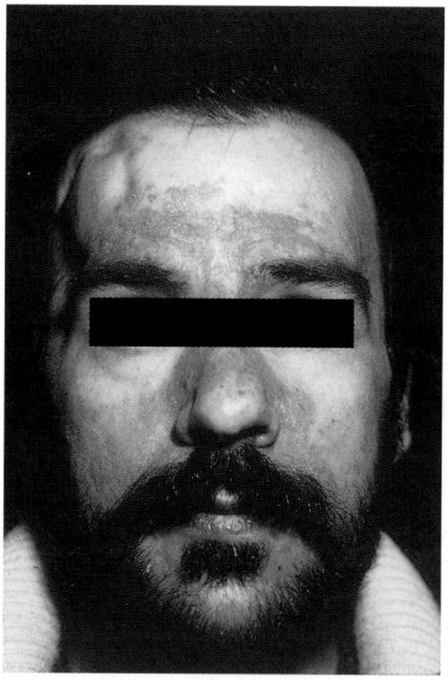

Fig. 19. Seborrhoeic dermatitis: inflammatory, erythematous and scaling eruption on the face

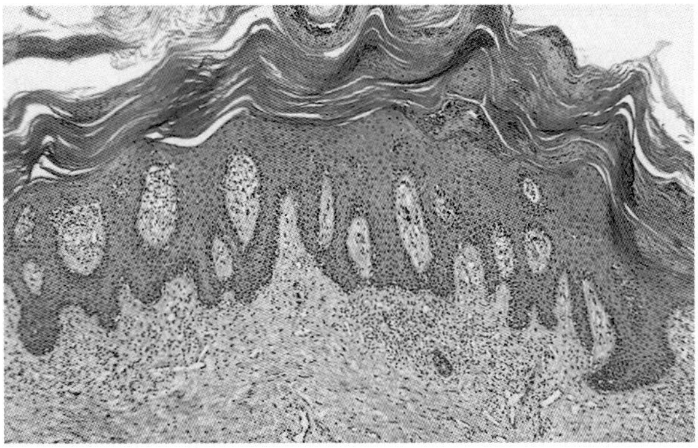

Fig. 20. Seborrhoeic dermatitis: irregular psoriasiform hyperplasia of the epidermis

P. ovale in SD of HIV is due to an altered cellular immunity probably induced by increased IL-10 secretion [80]. HIV-infected patients with low CD4 counts had more severe SD [81], but it is not thought to be associated with a poor prognosis [82]. Isolated aspects of SD have occasionally been reported as early signs of HIV infection [83]. The histopathological findings of SD are similar to those seen in patients with non-HIV-associated disease. The early lesions show a "basket-weave" cornified layer and a superficial perivascular lymphohistiocytic infiltrate with plasma cells. Exocytosis of lymphocytes in the epidermis and scattered necrotic keratinocytes are often present. Sharply defined small lymphocyte clusters obliterate the dermo-epidermal junction in a minority of cases. Blood vessels of the superficial plexus are dilated and a few extravasated erythrocytes are present in the dermal papillae. The more developed lesions are characterised by extensive parakeratosis with neutrophils and plasma, as well as irregular psoriasiform hyperplasia of the epidermis (Fig. 20). Many lymphocytes are present singly throughout the epidermis, but scattered necrotic keratinocytes are less evident (Fig. 21). The perivascular infiltrate extends more deeply into the mid and deep dermis. In addition to numerous plasma cells, a few neutrophils are also present. Fragments of nuclear dust are scattered between the inflammatory cells, and the

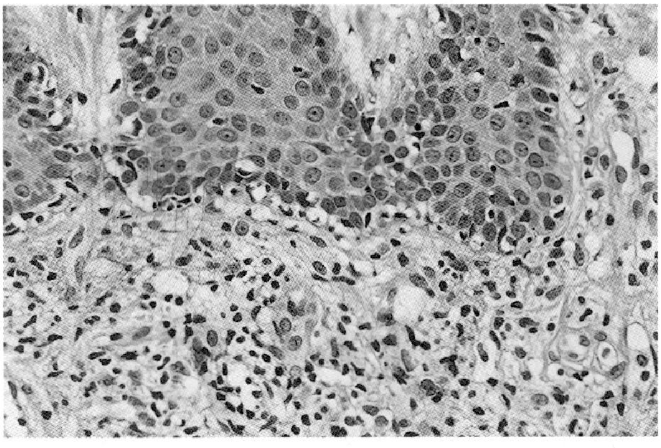

Fig. 21. Seborrhoeic dermatitis: lymphocytes are present throughout the epidermis

capillaries often show thick walls. Vasculitis is not noted. The follicular ostia are often dilated and plugged by hyperkeratosis. Long-standing lesions show a thin, hyperkeratotic epidermis. A perivascular lymphocytic infiltrate with plasma cells continues to be noted, although to a lesser degree, and follicular plugging remains prominent.

6.2 Psoriasis

Infection with HIV is associated with psoriasis with an incidence similar to that in the general population (1%–2%); nevertheless, psoriasis in HIV-infected patients may show marked exacerbations, may be one of the first manifestations of HIV disease, or may signal disease progression [84, 85]. The aetiological mechanisms remain unclear, but the condition is most likely due to a combination of genetic and environmental factors [84, 85]. Clinically, the lesions are similar to those seen in the immunocompetent host, resulting in an inverse pattern, with prominent plaques in the scalp, axillae and groin reported when HIV infection preceded the onset of psoriasis. Although psoriasis is often viewed, also in HIV-infected patients, as a disease without serious sequelae, severe variants such as the erythrodermic and generalised pustular types may be associated with serious morbidity and mortality [86].

Histologically, the characteristic findings of psoriasis can be observed in only a minority of these patients. Psoriasiform hyperplasia is seen, often with more irregular acanthosis, less suprapapillary thinning of the epidermis, poorly formed spongiform pustules, and a lymphoplasmacytic infiltrate in the dermis. The recognition of numerous plasma cells in psoriatic lesions should alert the pathologist to the possibility of HIV infection.

6.3 Reiter's Syndrome

Reiter's syndrome was first described in association with HIV in 1987. It is reported in 6%–10% of HIV-infected patients, being, with other reactive arthritides, the most common arthritis seen in AIDS patients [87].

Clinically, Reiter's syndrome is defined as an episode of peripheral arthritis of more than 1 month duration occurring in association with urethritis and/or cervicitis [88]. Nevertheless, cutaneous manifestations are also reported in half of affected patients, such as pustular or papular lesions of the glabrous skin, glans penis (balanitis circinata) and scalp. Also hyperkeratosis and shedding of the nail plate are described. The course of Reiter's syndrome is more severe, progressive and refractory to treatment in HIV patients than in non-HIV-positive patients. The aetiological mechanism remains unclear but most likely it is a combination of genetic and environmental factors [89]. The decrease of CD4 lymphocytes, the increase of CD8 lymphocytes and the modification of immune regulation may be important in the pathogenesis [90]. The histopathological picture is that of a pustular psoriasis with the characteristic spongiform pustule of Kogoj. Early pustular lesions appear as spongiform macropustules in the upper epidermis with parakeratosis and elongation of the rete ridges. In the oldest lesions the parakeratotic cornified layer overlying the spongiform pustule thickens considerably and consists of parakeratotic cells intermingled with the picmotic nuclei of neutrophils.

6.4 Prurigo Nodularis

Prurigo nodularis (PN) is a reaction pattern that may be associated with many underlying causes of itching. It is characterised by intensely itchy nodules which are classically localised in symmetric fashion mainly to the limbs and sometimes affect the trunk. The cause is unknown. Not all patients with pruritus develop PN, and this is because there may be a familial predisposition to its development; nevertheless, pruritus is requisite for the development of PN. In AIDS patients, one of the most common causes of itching is a response to an arthropod bite. In addition, in HIV-infected patients there are other pruritic dermatoses that may result in the development of PN, such as eosinophilic folliculitis and scabies. Systemic causes of generalised pruritus, such as neoplasms – especially lymphoma, anaemia, hepatic dysfunction and renal disease, reported in immunocompetent patients also may be the causes of PN in HIV infection [91].

Clinically, numerous discrete, intensely itchy pink or brown papules and nodules are seen, located on the extremities and on the trunk. They are excoriated and healed white scars which sometimes have very obvious follicular openings within them. A perilesional postinflammatory pigmentary alteration consistent with hypo- and/or hyperpigmented macules and patches is often present [92].

Histologically, the main features are pronounced hyperkeratosis and irregular acanthosis. Occasionally papillomatosis and irregular downward proliferation of the epidermis and adnexal epithelium may be observed, similar to pseudocarcinomatous hyperplasia. The papillary dermis presents a predominantly lymphocytic inflammatory infiltrate and collagen bundles orientated parallel to elongated epidermal retia. Occasionally, hyperplasia of nerve twigs in the upper dermis may be observed; however, this is an uncommon finding and is not considered by some authors to be an essential feature for the diagnosis of PN. In some cases, silver stains or cholinesterase stains demonstrate an increased number of cutaneous nerves. Eosinophils, mast cells and basophils are occasionally present in the epidermis and dermis. A marked eosinophil degranulation may be seen more frequently in patients with an atopic background [93].

6.5 Eosinophilic Folliculitis

Eosinophilic folliculitis (EF) is a pruritic dermatosis that nearly always develops in patient with CD4 lymphocyte counts below 200 cells/mm^3. This condition is an important marker of advanced HIV infection. It was originally described in 1970 by Ofuji in an adult Japanese patient. The condition is now known to be geographically more widespread and may be seen in children.

The pathogenesis of the disorder is not fully known but it is thought to be secondary to normally innocuous follicular antigens becoming antigenic in a Th2-dominant milieu. In fact, a pemphigus-like antibody involving the lower portion of the epidermis has been demonstrated, and an antibody directed against the cytoplasm of the basal cells of the outer root sheath of follicles has also been reported. Neutrophil and eosinophil chemotactic factors in stratum corneum extracts from lesions have also been demonstrated. Activation of cell adhesion molecule expression may be involved in the selective migration of eosinophils and lymphocytes into the involved hair follicle epithelium [16].

Clinically, patients develop folliculocentric pruritic urticarial papules measuring 1–4 mm in diameter, most commonly on the upper trunk, face, neck and proximal extremities. It appears similar to a number of other pruritic dermatoses that may be found in HIV-infected individuals as well as in bacterial folliculitis, insect bite reactions, scabies and dermatitis herpetiformis [94].

Histologically, involved follicles may show spongiotic change with exocytosis extending from the sebaceous gland and its duct throughout the infundibular zone. Lymphocytes with some eosinophils migrate into the epidermis initially in a somewhat diffuse pattern, but micropustular aggregation develops and the ultimate result is infundibular eosinophilic pustules. When follicles rupture, there is an intense perifollicular inflammatory infiltrate with marked perifollicular fibrosis [95].

6.6 Xerotic Dermatitis

Dry skin has been reported in some AIDS patients and represents a condition of advanced disease. It may be the port of entry for secondary infection of fungi and bacteria. It is notable that other conditions where the immune system is altered, such as Hodgkin's lymphoma, lepromatous leprosy, and sarcoidosis, may present as acquired ichthyosis [96].

6.7 Porphyria Cutanea Tarda

Since Wissel's mention of the first three cases in 1987, many cases of HIV-associated porphyria cutanea tarda (PCT) have been reported [97] PCT can reveal HIV infection, although it occurs late, at the B or C stage (CDC 1993) with $CD4^+$ T lymphocytes almost always below 200/mm^3. There is a strong association between PCT and hepatitis C virus (HCV). As HIV and HCV infection have common risk factors, especially blood transfusion and intravenous drug abuse, HIV-associated PCT might also be related to HCV. These co-factors are probably triggers for the appearance of PCT in HIV-positive patients [98].

Clinically we see blisters on sun-exposed areas, especially the hands, with crusting, milia formation, dyspigmentation and scarring. Malar areas of the face present hyperpigmentation and hypertrichosis. The urine is often dark [99].

The histopathological aspect is similar to that seen in immunocompetent patients and shows a subepidermal blister (Fig. 22) with minimal inflammation in

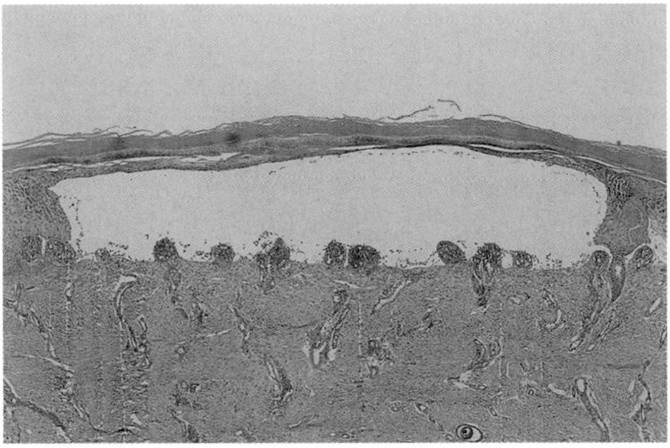

Fig. 22. Porphyria cutanea tarda: subepidermal bulla

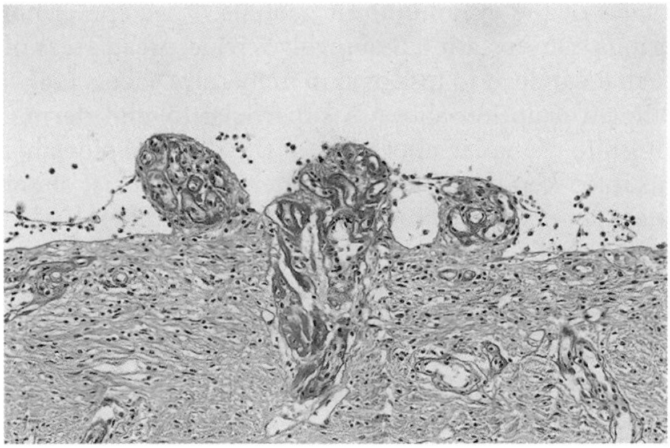

Fig. 23. Porphyria cutanea tarda: preservation of dermal papillae (so-called festooning) at the base of the bulla

the dermis, and a direct immunofluorescence study reveals perivascular deposition of immunoglobulins and complement. Elongated aggregations of necrotic keratinocytes are often present in the epidermis, overlying the blister, and have been referred to as "caterpillar bodies". Preservation of dermal papillae – so-called festooning (Fig. 23) – is seen, and there are thick, hyaline PAS-positive rims surrounding blood vessels in the upper dermis. The diagnosis of PCT is based on clinical appearance, histological findings and discovery of elevated urinary uroporphyrins and coproporphyrins [16].

6.8 Cutaneous Drug Eruptions

Drug hypersensitivity reactions occur commonly in patients with HIV [100]. Hypersensitivity is significantly more common in patients with HIV infection than in those with other immunodeficiency disorders or in the general population [101]. The causes and mechanisms of this hypersensitivity are not known, but they are likely to include a high dose or prolonged duration of therapy, the degree of immunodeficiency, glutathione deficiency, and perhaps coexisting viral infection or immune complex deposition [102, 103].

Trimethoprim-sulfamethoxazole is the best known and most common drug causing a cutaneous eruption in patients with HIV infection. Other antibiotics that commonly induce drug eruption in these patients include isoniazid, clathomicin, rifampicin and amoxicillin and clavulonic acid. As in the general population, a morbilliform rash is the most common type of drug-related eruption in HIV-infected patients. It is characterised by a widespread eruption of fine pink to red macules and papules involving the extremities that develops 8–12 days after therapy is initiated, reaching maximal intensity 1–2 days later. In some cases, desquamation may supervene. The eruption may disappear within 3–5 days even though therapy is continued, although in some cases it may persist for days to weeks following discontinuation of the medication. Stevens-Johnson syndrome, urticaria, erythema multiforme and toxic epidermal necrolysis may also develop. Stevens-Johnson syndrome is characterised by fever with widespread blistering of the skin and mucous membranes of the eye, mouth or genitals. Toxic epidermal necrolysis (TEN) is a more serious manifestation that involves widespread areas of the skin with confluent bullae that can lead to loss of skin in massive sheets [16].

Histologically, the morbilliform eruption shows a superficial to mid-dermal perivascular mononuclear infiltrate, vacuolar alteration of the dermo-epidermal junction and individually necrotic keratinocytes. Prominent spongiosis, slight parakeratosis and scattered plasma cells may occasionally be observed [16, 104].

Some authors have reported cases of foscarnet ulcers as a consequence of direct toxicity of the agent on the mucous membrane. Some cases of hyperpigmentation have been related to AZT therapy, although the condition is also reported in HIV-infected patients who have never been given AZT [105].

Protease inhibitor treatment has dramatically improved the morbidity and mortality in HIV-infected patients. Recently, a number of syndromes have been described involving abnormal fat distribution that may be associated with prolonged HIV-protease inhibitor therapy. These include hypertrophy of the cervicodorsal fat pad ("buffalo hump"); a tendency toward increased central adiposity ("protease paunch"); adiposity in the submental, mandibular, and lateral cheek regions of the face; and hypertrophy of adipose tissue in the breast in women. A peripheral lipodistrophy, or fat-wasting, in the extremities and face (particularly the malar and nasolabial fold regions) has also been observed: As these patients live longer and healthier lives, many are beginning to seek surgical correction of the disfigurements [106]. Other adverse dermatological effects of HAART such us alopecia, dry skin, pruritic skin eruptions and paronychia have been reported as well [107–109].

6.9 Hair and Nail Abnormalities

Some cases of alopecia universalis are reported in HIV-positive patients, often associated with decreased $CD4^+$ counts [16]; premature greying, thinning, and hair loss may also occur. Nail deformities have been reported in patients with AIDS. Some patients develop a yellow discoloration of the distal portion of the nail.

Transverse or longitudinal ridging of the nails may occur. Loss or decrease in size of the lunula and opaqueness with or without onycholysis may also be seen [110].

7 AIDS-Related Malignancies

Worldwide, it is estimated that about 33.4 million people are currently infected with HIV. There have been about 16,000 new infections daily during the past year. By some estimates, up to 40% of patients with AIDS will ultimately develop some form of cancer [111]. Despite advances in antiretroviral therapy and in the treatment and prevention of opportunistic infections, oncological and consequent haematological complications of HIV infection continue to occur and are of significant clinical importance. Virus-related tumours (e.g., Kaposi's sarcoma, induced by human herpes virus 8; non-Hodgkin's lymphoma, linked to Epstein-Barr virus; and anogenital tumours linked to human papillomavirus) are frequent in patients with HIV-induced immune deficiency [112]. In addition, several reports suggest that a number of other malignancies may occur at an increased incidence in persons with HIV infection, including squamous-cell carcinoma of the head, neck and anus, plasmacytoma, melanoma, small-cell lung cancer, basal-cell carcinoma, and germ-cell tumours [113]. Melanomas among patients with HIV infection are often atypical in appearance, being multiple or metastatic as is the case in other well-defined immunosuppressed groups [114]. Clinicians and pathologists should become familiar with HIV-related malignancies, as their incidence is expected to further increase as more effective therapies for HIV and associated opportunistic infections allow patients to live longer in an advanced state of immunodeficiency [115].

7.1 Lymphomas

Non-Hodgkin's lymphomas are more common in patients with AIDS than in the general population and they occur in about 10% of HIV-infected patients. They also differ from those observed in immunocompetent patients in relation to their location, histology, natural history and response to treatment. The lymphoid system is doubly affected in AIDS, being the target both of the initial viral infection that produces the immune deficiency and of the second viral infection that produces neoplasia [116].

In HIV patients the risk of developing a malignant lymphoma is calculated to be between 60 and 100 times greater than that expected in the general population and it represents a late manifestation of HIV infection. In fact, the incidence of lymphoma increases with prolonged survival in patients, probably due to effective antiretroviral therapy [117].

AIDS lymphomas differ from those occurring in the general population, being predominantly high-grade non-Hodgkin's lymphomas. They show a notable tendency to present at extranodal sites and are usually derived from B cells (Fig. 24) [118, 119].

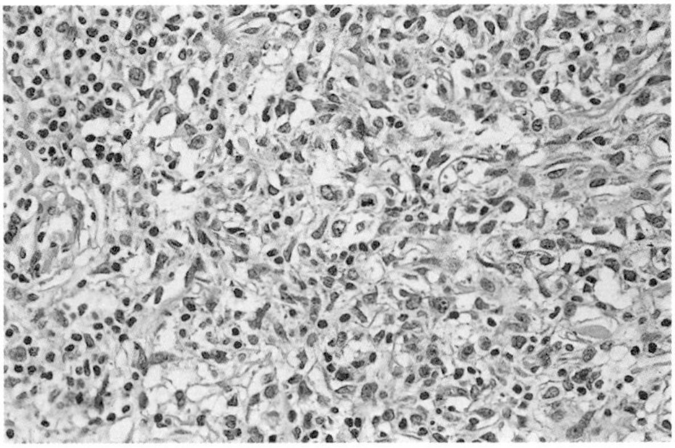

Fig. 24. Lymphoma: large anaplastic B-cell lymphoma with mitotic figures

Cutaneous non-Hodgkin's lymphomas are rare in patients with HIV infection and almost all of the cases reported are of T-cell lineage with histopathological features of mycosis fungoides or Sézary syndrome. A few cases of T-cell neoplasms are large non-Hodgkin lymphomas without epidermotropism [120, 121].

Cutaneous non-Hodgkin's lymphoma clinically appears either as a diffuse eruption of papules and/or nodules or as panniculitis. Papules or plaques similar to those observed in mycosis fungoides are also reported in T-cell lymphomas of HIV-infected patients. HTLV1-associated lymphomas having the clinical aspect of acute viral exanthema have been also described in these patients.

Cutaneous T-cell lymphoma can be histologically characterised by psoriasiform hyperplasia of the epidermis with a band-like infiltrate of atypical lymphocytes having cerebriform nuclei that are also present in the epidermis, where they often form small collections of microabscesses. A diffuse monomorphous infiltrate that involves the lower portion of the dermis and subcutaneous fat and spares the overlying epidermis can be occasionally seen. Atypical lymphoid cells that show a large and pleomorphic nucleus with mitosis are present.

The immunophenotype of mycosis fungoides-like cutaneous T-cell lymphoma in HIV patients is usually characterised by an infiltrate of $CD8^+$ lymphocytes, but it may be comprised of monoclonal $CD4^+$ cells [16].

7.2 Kaposi's Sarcoma

Kaposi's sarcoma is well known as the most frequently occurring malignant tumour in HIV-infected individuals, often leading to death [122]. The proportion of lethal outcomes in HIV-infected patients attributable to Kaposi's sarcoma is increasing, maybe as the result of combined antiretroviral therapy and better prophylaxis of opportunistic infection.

Kaposi's sarcoma is clinically classified on the basis of morphological presentation and biological behaviour and is divided into four types: benign-nodular, aggressive-infiltrative, florid, and lymphadenopathic [123].

Nodular Kaposi's sarcoma is a localised cutaneous disease. Infiltrative Kaposi's sarcoma is an aggressive cutaneous disease that may invade the underlying soft tissue and bone. Florid Kaposi's sarcoma is a widespread disease with mucocutaneous and visceral involvement. Lymphadenopathic Kaposi's sarcoma is a virulent form seen in prepubescent black African children [124].

The epidemiological classification of Kaposi's sarcoma includes sporadic or classical, endemic or African, epidemic or HIV-related, and iatrogenic or immunosuppression-associated [123]. Many studies have been performed to identify an infective agent in Kaposi's sarcoma. Human herpes virus 8 (HHV8) is so far the only agent found consistently in all forms of this disease. It was found in 94% cases of classical Kaposi's sarcoma, 100% of post-transplant Kaposi's sarcoma, 87% of endemic Kaposi's sarcoma and 100% of HIV-negative gay men with Kaposi's sarcoma [123]. It is possible that HHV8 acts indirectly, by triggering the release of cytokines expressed in Kaposi's sarcoma tissue and thus promoting the growth of Kaposi spindle cells in vivo. Kaposi's sarcoma itself may cause progressive immunosuppression through the interaction of HIV and HHV-8, which probably occurs in multiple ways. As in other acute or chronic infection [125], HHV-8 may accelerate HIV disease progression in co-infected individuals through interaction with the HIV co-receptors [125]. On the other hand, the HIV Tat protein seems to increase the HHV-8 viral load and may reactivate HHV-8 from a latent state [125].

Sporadic Kaposi's sarcoma occurs in the elderly, mainly in an acral distribution; they usually present with nodular cutaneous lesions that are slowly progressive. Sometimes they develop lymphedema and nodal involvement. Endemic Kaposi occurs mainly in areas of Africa; prior to the HIV epidemic it presented clinically with nodular or infiltrative Kaposi's sarcoma as well as lymphadenopathy in children. However, with HIV infection, patients in areas of the world with endemic Kaposi's sarcoma may develop features that are atypical and more consistent with florid Kaposi's sarcoma clinically [123]. Epidemic Kaposi's sarcoma occurs in HIV patients: homosexual men have the highest incidence, suggesting a plausible spread of the agent sexually [123]. The first lesions are pink macules and patches; in time papules appear, and dark nodules distributed mainly on the legs and feet. The lesions may coalesce to form large confluent plaques or tumours. On the other hand, every part may be involved: mucous membranes such as the hard palate, lips, penis, and nose, the trunk, and the scalp (Fig. 25).

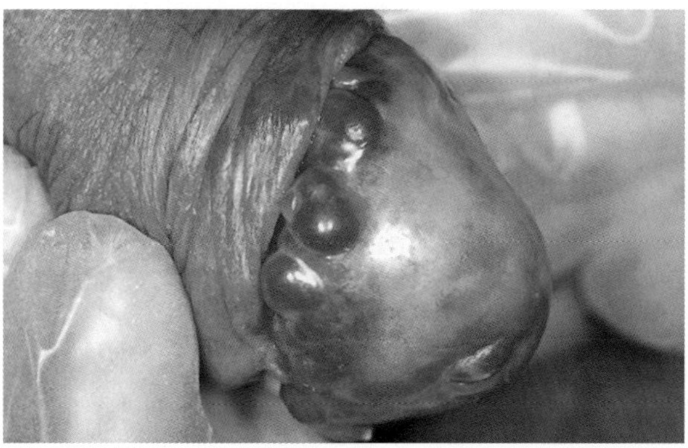

Fig. 25. Kaposi's sarcoma: Kaposi's sarcoma of the penis

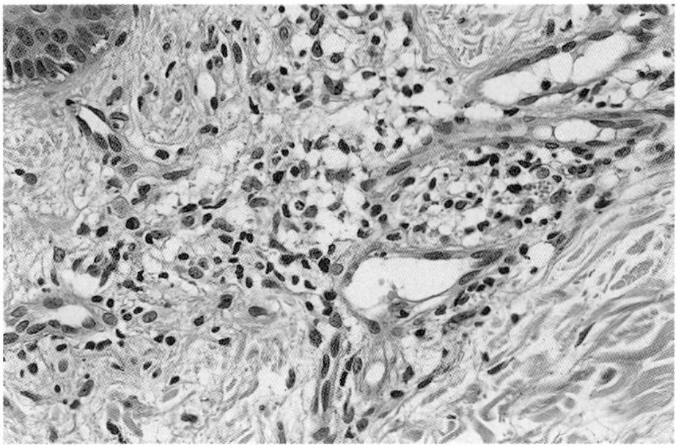

Fig. 26. Kaposi's sarcoma: small, irregular endothelial-line spaces with inflammatory infiltrate of lymphocytes

Histologically, Kaposi's sarcoma is a complex lesion varying in its clinical appearance. In early Kaposi's lesions, there is a collection of small, irregular endothelial-line spaces that surround normal dermal blood vessels, and these are accompanied by a variable, inflammatory infiltrate of lymphocytes (patch stage) (Fig. 26). This stage is followed by the expansion of a spindle-celled vascular process throughout the dermis. These spindle cells form slit-like vascular channels containing erythrocytes (plaque stage) (Fig. 27). In the later nodular stage, Kaposi's sarcoma lesions are composed of sheets of spindle cells, some of which are undergoing mitosis, and a slit-like vascular space with areas of haemosiderin pigmentation. The spindle cells form the bulb of established Kaposi's sarcoma lesions and are therefore thought to be the neoplastic component (Fig. 28), but some controversy still exists over the histogenesis of spindle cells. Although the majority of the spindle cells stain positive for endothelial cell markers, including factor VIII and CD34, some cells express proteins characteristic of smooth muscle cells, macrophages or dendritic cells [126, 127]. Circulating Kaposi's sarcoma-like spindle cells have been isolated and cultured from patients with AIDS-Kaposi's sarcoma and from those thought for other reasons to be at risk of AIDS-Kaposi's sarcoma [128]. These circulating cells have an adherent phenotype and express markers of both macrophage and endothelial cells [129].

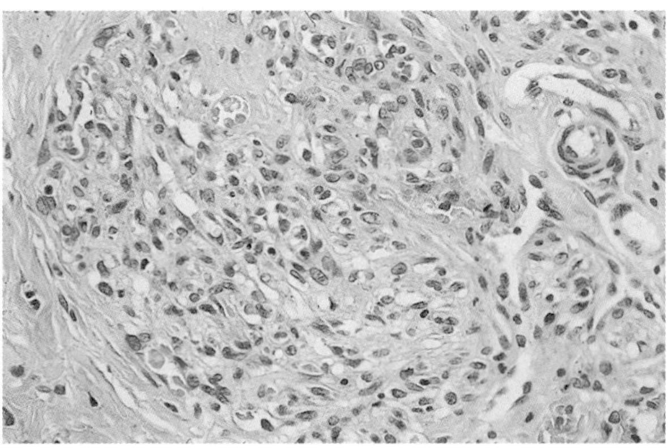

Fig. 27. Kaposi's sarcoma: vascular proliferation containing erythrocytes and haemosiderin granules

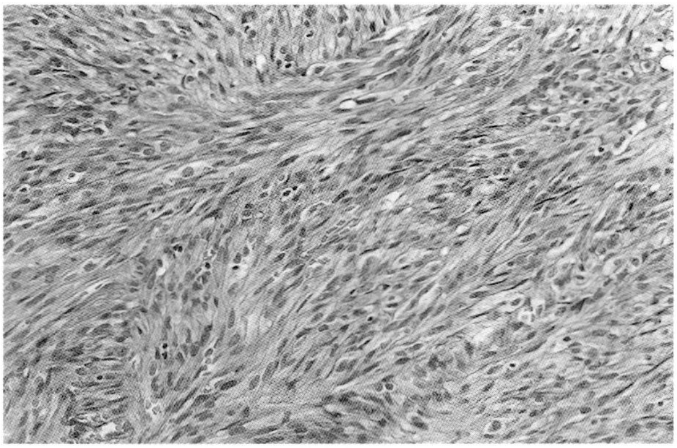

Fig. 28. Kaposi's sarcoma: spindle cells with mitosis in sarcomatous arrangement

Many different cutaneous disorders such as inflammatory and neoplastic conditions may simulate Kaposi's sarcoma. Clinically, purpura, haemangiomata, bacillary angiomatosis, dermatofibromata, lichen planus, pityriasis rosea, mycosis fungoides, naevi, malignant melanoma, cutaneous lymphoma, and secondary syphilis have all been reported as simulators of Kaposi's sarcoma.

Histologically, there are a number of different patterns that are similar to Kaposi's sarcoma findings. Some of these include microvenular haemangioma, targetoid haemosiderotic haemangioma, proliferative angiomata, severe stasis dermatitis, granuloma annulare and dermatofibroma.

References

1. Mertens TE, Low-Beer D (1996) HIV and AIDS: where is the epidemic going? Bull World Health Organ 74:121–129
2. Tschachler E, Bergstresser PR, Stingl G (1996) HIV-related skin diseases. Lancet 348: 659–663
3. McCullough MJ, Firth NA, Reade PC (1997) Human immunodeficiency virus infection: a review of the mode of infection, pathogenesis, disease course and the general and clinical manifestations. Australian Dental J 42:30–37
4. Romagnani S (1995) Biology of human Th1 and Th2 cells. J Clin Immunol 15:121–129
5. Barnadas MA, Alegre M, Baselga E, Randazzo L, Margall N, Rabella N, Curell R, de Moragas JM (1997) Histopathological changes of primary HIV infection. Description of three cases and review of literature. J Cutan Pathol 24:507–510
6. Hulsebosch HJ, Claessen FA, van Ginkel CJ, Kuiters GR, Goudsmit J, Lange JM (1990) Human immunodeficiency virus exanthem. J Am Acad Dermatol 23:483–486
7. Brehemer-Andersson E, Torssander J (1990) The exanthema of acute (primary) HIV infection. Identification of a characteristic histopathological picture? Acta Derm Venereol 70:85–87
8. Balslev E, Thomsen HK, Weismann K (1990) Histopathology of acute human immunodeficiency virus exanthema. J Clin Pathol 43:201–202
9. Warner LC, Fisher BK (1986) Cutaneous manifestations of the acquired immunodeficiency syndrome. Int J Dermatol 25:337–350
10. Langtry JA, Ostlere LS, Hawkins DA, Staughton RC (1994) The difficulty in diagnosis of cutaneous herpes simplex virus infection in patients with AIDS. Clin Exp Dermatol 19:224–226
11. Tyring SK, Carlton SS, Evans T (1998) Herpes atypical clinical manifestations. Dermatol Clin 16:783–788

12. Griffiths PD (1996) Herpesviruses and AIDS. Scand J Infect Dis 100 [Suppl]: 3–7
13. Garcia-Plata MD, Moreno-Gimenez JC, Velez-Garcia A, Valverde Blanco F, Fernandez Roldan JC (1999) Herpetic whitlow in an AIDS patient. J Eur Acad Dermatol Venereol 12:241–242
14. Lokke Jensen B, Weismann K, Mathiesen L, Klem Thomsen H (1993) Atypical varicella-zoster infection in AIDS. Acta Derm Venereol 73:123–125
15. Hoppenjans WB, Bibler MR, Orme RL, Solinger AM (1990) Prolonged cutaneous herpes zoster in acquired immunodeficiency syndrome. Arch Dermatol 126:1048–1050
16. Aftergut K, Cockerell C (1999) Update on the cutaneous manifestations of HIV infection. Dermatol Clin 17:445–471
17. Blankenship W, Herchline T, Hockley A (1994) Asymptomatic vesicles in a patient with the acquired immunodeficiency syndrome. Disseminated varicella-zoster virus (VZV) infection. Arch Dermatol 130:1193–1196
18. LeBoit PE, Limova M, Yen TS, Palefsky JM, White CR jr, Berger TG (1992) Chronic verrucous varicella-zoster virus infection in patients with the acquired immunodeficiency syndrome (AIDS). Histologic and molecular biologic findings. Am J Dermatopathol 14:1–7
19. Vaughan Jones SA, McGibbon DH, Bradbeer CS (1994) Chronic verrucous varicella-zoster infection in a patient with AIDS. Clin Exp Dermatol 19:327–329
20. Greenberg MS (1996) HIV-associated lesions. Dermatol Clin 14:319–326
21. Bournerias I, Boismic S, Patey O, et al. (1989) Unusual cutaneous cytomegalovirus involvement in patients with acquired immunodeficiency syndrome. Arch Dermatol 125:1243–1246
22. Triantos D, Porter SR, Scully C, Teo CG (1997) Oral hairy leukoplakia: clinicopathologic features, pathogenesis, diagnosis and clinical significance. Clin Infect Dis 25:1392–1396
23. Guccion JG, Redman RS (1999) Oral hairy leukoplakia: an ultrastructural study and review of the literature. Ultrastruct Pathol 23:181–187
24. Brehemer-Andersson E, Lucht E, Lindskog S, Ekman M, Biberfeld P (1994) Oral hairy leukoplakia: pathogenetic aspects and significance of the lesion. Acta Derm Venereol 74:81–89
25. Chopra KF, Tyring SK (1997) The impact of the human immunodeficiency virus on the human papillomavirus epidemic. Arch Dermatol 133:629–633
26. de Villiers EM (1994) Human pathogenic papillomavirus types: an update. Curr Top Micriobiol 186:1–12
27. Lorincz AT, Reid R, Jenson AB, et al. (1992) Human papillomavirus infection of the cervix: relative risk associations of 15 common anogenital types. Obstet Gynecol 79:328–337
28. Fazel N, Wilczynski S, Lowe L, Su LD (1999) Clinical, histopathologic, and molecular aspects of cutaneous human papillomavirus infections. Dermatol Clin 17:521–536
29. Meberg R, Kenyon E, Bierman R, Loveland L, Barbosa P (1998) Characterization of plantar verrucae among individuals with human immunodeficiency virus. J Am Podiatr Med Assoc 88:442–445
30. Jablonska S, Dabrowski J, Jakubowicz K (1972) Epidermodysplasia verruciformis as a model in studies on the role of papillomaviruses in oncogenesis. Cancer Res 32:583–589
31. Berger TG, Sawchuk WS, Leonardi C et al. (1991) Epidermodysplasia verruciformis-associated Papillomavirus infection complicating human immunodeficiency virus disease. Br J Dermatol 124:79–83
32. LeBoit PE (1992) Dermatopathologic findings in patients infected with HIV. Dermatol Clin 10:59–71
33. Sykes NL Jr. Condyloma acuminatum. Int J Dermatol (1995) 34:297–302
34. Wade TR, Kopf AW, Ackerman AB (1978) Bowenoid papulosis of the penis. Cancer 42:1890–903
35. Waugh MA (1998) Molluscum contagiosum. Dermatol Clin 16:839–841
36. Petersen CS, Gerstoft (1992) Molluscum contagiosum in HIV-infected patients. J Clin Lab Inv 184:19–21
37. Scully M, Berger TG (1990) Pruritus, Staphylococcus aureus, and human immunodeficiency virus infection. Arch Dermatol 126:684–685

38. Becker BA, Frieden IJ, Odom RB, Berger TG (1989) Atypical plaquelike staphylococcal folliculitis in human immunodeficiency virus-infected persons. J Am Acad Dermatol 21:1024–1026
39. Richard M, Mathieu-Serra A (1986) Staphylococcal scalded skin syndrome in a homosexual adult. J Am Acad Dermatol 15:385–389
40. Kline MW, Dunkle LM (1988) Toxic shock syndrome and the acquired immunodeficiency syndrome. Pediatr Infect Dis 10:736–738
41. Stoler MH, Bonfiglio TA, Steigbigel RT, et al. (1983) An atypical subcutaneous infection associated with acquired immunodeficiency syndrome. Am J Clin Pathol 80:714–718
42. Bachelez H, Oksenhendler E, Lebbé C, Dauga C, Pinquier L, Mainguene C, Clauvel JP, Grimont PAD, Morel P, Dubertret L, Arlet G (1995) Bacillary angiomatosis in HIV-infected patients: report of three cases with different clinical courses and identification of Rochalimaea quintana as the aetiological agent. Br J Dermatol 133:983–989
43. Innocenzi D, Cerio R, Barduagni O, Bosman C, Carlesimo OA (1993) Bacillary epithelioid angiomatosis in acquired immunodeficiency syndrome (AIDS) – clinicopathological and ultrastructural study of a case with a review of the literature. Clin Exp Dermatol 18:133–137
44. Moroni M, Gori A, Rusconi S, Franzetti F, Antinori S (1994) Mycobacterial infections in AIDS: an overview of epidemiology, clinical manifestations, therapy and prophylaxis. Monaldi Arch Chest Dis 49:432–438
45. Porter JD (1996) Mycobacteriosis and HIV infection: the new public health challenge. J Antimicrob Chemother 37 [Suppl B]: 113–120
46. Quinn TC, Common RO, Glasser D, et al. (1990) The association of syphilis with the risk of human immunodeficiency virus infection in patients attending sexually transmitted disease clinics. Arch Intern Med 50:1297–1302
47. Pappas PG (1993) Syphilis 100 years ago: parallels with the AIDS pandemic. Int J Dermatol 32:708–709
48. Glover RA, Piaquadio DJ, Kern S, Cockerell CJ (1992) An unusual presentation of secondary syphilis in a patient with human immunodeficiency virus infection. A case report and review of the literature. Arch Dermatol 128:530–534
49. Engelkens HJ, van der Sluis JJ, Stolz E (1991) Syphilis in the AIDS era. Int J Dermatol 30:254–256
50. Bitman LM, Rabinowitz AD (1998) Hyperkeratotic plantar plaques in an HIV-positive patient. Crusted scabies, localized to the soles. Arch Dermatol 134:1019, 1022–1023
51. Guggisberg D, de Viragh PA, Constantin C, Panizzon RG (1998) Norwegian scabies in a patient with acquired immunodeficiency syndrome. Dermatology 197:306–308
52. Orkin M (1993) Scabies in AIDS. Semin Dermatol 12:9–14
53. Bartlett JG (1998) Natural history and classification. In: Bartlett JG (ed) Medical management of HIV infection. Johns Hopkins University, Baltimore, Maryland, pp 1–16
54. Lapins J, Lindback S, Lidbrink P, Biberfeld P, Emtestam L, Gaines H (1996) Mucocutaneous manifestations in 22 consecutive cases of primary HIV-1 infection. Br J Dermatol 134: 257–261
55. Disler RS, Dover JS (1990) Chronic localized herpes zoster in the acquired immunodeficiency syndrome. Arch Dermatol 126:1105–1106
56. Wright SW, Johnson RA (1997) Human immunodeficiency virus in women: mucocutaneous manifestations. Clin Dermatol 15:93–111
57. Penneys N (1997) Disease caused by viruses. In: Elder D, Elenitsas R, Jaworsky C, et al. (eds) Lever's histopathology of the skin, 8th edn. Lippincott-Raven, Philadelphia, p 578
58. Weedon D (1997) Viral diseases. In: Weedon D, Strutton G (eds) Skin pathology. Churchill-Livingstone, Edinburgh, p 592
59. Northfelt DW, Palefsky JM (1992) Human papillomavirus-associated anogenital neoplasia in persons with HIV infection. AIDS Clin Rev 44:241–259
60. Gerber GS (1994) Carcinoma in situ of the penis. J Urol 151:829–833
61. Wade TR, Kopf AW, Ackerman AB (1978) Bowenoid papulosis of the penis. Cancer 42:1890–1903
62. Curry A, Turner AJ, Lucas S (1991) Opportunistic protozoan infections in human immunodeficiency virus disease: review highlighting diagnostic and therapeutic aspects. J Clin Pathol 44:182–193

63. Litwin MA, Williams CM (1992) Cutaneous Pneumocystis carinii infection mimicking Kaposi's sarcoma. Ann Intern Med 117:48–49
64. Hennessey NP, Parro EL, Cockerell CJ (1991) Cutaneous Pneumocystis carinii infection in patients with acquired immunodeficiency syndrome. Arch Dermatol 127:1699–1701
65. Hennessey NP, Cockerell CJ (1991) Cutaneous Pneumocystis carinii infection in patients with AIDS. Int Conf AIDS 7:241
66. Elmets CA (1994) Management of common superficial fungal infections in patients with AIDS. J Am Acad Dermatol 31:S60–S63
67. McCarthy GM, Mackie ID, Koval J, et al. (1991) Factors associated with increased frequency of HIV-related oral candidiasis. J Oral Pathol Med 20:332
68. Samaranayaka LP (1992) Oral mycoses in HIV infection. Oral Surg Oral Med Oral Pathol 73:171
69. Greenspan D (1994) Treatment of oropharingeal candidiasis in HIV-positive patients. J Am Acad Dermatol 31:S51–S55
70. Katz MH, Greenspan D, Westenhouse J, et al. (1992) Progression to AIDS in HIV-infected homosexual and bisexual men with hairy leukoplakia and oral candidiasis. AIDS 6:95
71. Odom RB (1994) Common superficial fungal infection in immunosuppressed patients. J Am Acad Dermatol 31:S56–S69
72. Cohen PR, Bank DE, Silver DN, et al. (1990) Cutaneous lesions of disseminated histoplasmosis in human immunodeficiency virus-infected patients. J Am Acad Dermatol 23:422–8
73. Cohen PR, Held JL, Grossman ME, et al. (1991) Disseminated histoplasmosis presenting as an ulcerated verrucous plaque in HIV-infected man. Int J Dermatol 30:104–108
74. Smith KJ, Skelton III HG, Angritt P (1991) Histopathologic features of HIV-associated skin disease. Dermatol Clin 9:551–577
75. Shahab ST, Habts-Gabr E, Fedorko D (1991) Significance of cryptococcal antigen titers in patients with AIDS. South Med J 84:1407–1408
76. Durden FM, Elewski B (1994) Cutaneous involvement of Cryptococcus neoformans in AIDS. JAAD 30:844–848
77. Wright DC, Lennox JL, James WD, et al. (1991) Generalized chronic dermatophytosis in patients with human immunodeficiency virus type I infection and CD 4 depletion. Arch Dermatol 127:265–266
78. Coldiron BM, Bergstresser PR (1989) Prevalence and clinical spectrum of skin disease in patients infected with human immunodeficiency virus. Arch Dermatol 125:357–361
79. Neuber K, Kroger S, Gruseck E, Abeck D, Ring J (1996) Effects of Pityrosporum ovale on proliferation, immunoglobulin (IgA, G, M) synthesis and cytokine (IL-2, IL-10, IFN gamma) production of peripheral blood mononuclear cells from patients with seborrheic dermatitis. Arch Dermatol Res 288:532–536
80. Schechtman RC, Midgley G, Hay RJ (1995) HIV disease and Malassezia yeasts: a quantitative study of patients presenting with seborrheic dermatitis. Br J Dermatol 133:694–698
81. Sindrup JH, Lisby G, Weisman K, et al. (1987) Skin manifestations of AIDS, HIV infection and ARC. Int J Dermatol 26:267–272
82. Mahè A, Boulais C, Blanc L et al. (1994) Seborrhoic dermatitis as a revealing feature of HIV infection in Bamako (Mali). Int J Dermatol 33:601–602
83. Soeprono FF, Schinella RA, Cockerell CJ, Comite SL (1986) Seborrheic-like dermatitis of acquired immunodeficiency syndrome. A clinicopathology study. J Am Acad Dermatol 14:242–248
84. Horn TD, Herzberg GZ, Hood AF (1990) Characterization of the dermal infiltrate in human immunodeficiency virus-infected patients with psoriasis. Arch Dermatol 126: 1462–1465
85. Wolfer LU, Djemadji-Oudjiel N, Hiletework M, Tebbe B, Husak R, Goerdt S, Orfanos CE (1998) HIV-associated psoriasis. Clinical and histological observations in 36 patients (in German). Hautarzt 49:197–202
86. Green MS, Prystowsky JH, Cohen SR, Cohen JI, Lebwohl MG (1996) Infectious complications of erythrodermic psoriasis. J Am Acad Dermatol 34:911–914
87. Kaye BR (1989) Rheumatologic manifestations of infection with human immunodeficiency virus (HIV). Ann Intern Med 111:158–167

88. Altman EM, Centeno LV, Mahal M, Bielory L (1994). AIDS-associated Reiter's sndrome. Ann Allergy 72:307–316
89. Weitzul S, Duvic M (1997) HIV-related psoriasis and Reiter's syndrome. Semin Cutan Med Surg 16:213–218
90. de Mello e Silva AC, Boulos M (1998) Reiter's syndrome and human immunodeficiency virus infection (in Portuguese). Rev Hosp Clin Fac Med Sao Paulo 53:202–204
91. Kundu A, Wade AA, Ilchyshyn A (1995) Prurigo nodularis in an HIV positive man. Genitourin Med 71:129–130
92. Matthews SN, Cockerell CJ (1998) Prurigo nodularis in HIV-infected individuals. Int J Dermatol 37:401–409
93. Mattila JO, Vornanen M, Katila ML (1997) Histopathological and bacteriological findings in prurigo nodularis. Acta Derm Venereol 77:49–51
94. Soeprono FF, Schinella RA (1986) Eosinophilic pustular folliculitis in patients with acquired immunodeficiency syndrome. Report of three cases. J Am Acad Dermatol 14:1020–1022
95. McCalmont TH, Altmus D, Maurer T, Berger TG (1995) Eosinophilic folliculitis. The histologic spectrum. Am J Dermatopathol 17:439–446
96. Warner LC, Benjamin K, Fisher (1986) Cutaneous manifestations of the acquired Immunodeficiency Syndrome. Int J Der 25:337–350
97. Blauvelt A (1996) Hepatitis C virus and human immunodeficiency virus infection can alter porphyrin metabolism and lead to porphyria cutanea tarda. Arch Dermatol 132:1503–1504
98. Wissel PS, Sordillo P, Anderson KE, Sassa S, Savillo RL, Kappas A (1987) Porphyria cutanea tarda associated with acquired immune deficiency syndrome. Am J Hematol 25:107–111
99. O'Connor W J, Murphy GM, Darby C, Fogarty J, Mulcahy F, O'Moore R, Barnes L (1996) Porphyrin abnormalities in acquired immunodeficiency syndrome. Arch Dermatol 132: 1443–1447
100. Carr A, Vasak E, Munro V, Penny R, Cooper DA (1994) Immunohistological assessment of cutaneous drug hypersensitivity in patients with HIV infection. Clin Exp Immunol 97:260–265
101. Coopman MA, Johnson RA, Platt R, Stern RS (1993) Cutaneous disease and drug reaction in HIV infection. N Engl J Med 328:1670–1674
102. Carr A, Cooper DA, Penny R (1991) Allergic manifestation of human immunodeficiency virus (HIV) infection. J Clin Immun 11:55–64
103. Carr A, Gross A, Hoskins J, Penny R, Cooper DA (1994) Acetylation phenotype and hypersensitivity to trimethoprin-sulphamethoxazole in HIV-infected patients. AIDS 8:333–337
104. Smith KJ, Skelton HG, Yeager J, Ledsky R, T-H NG, Wagner KF, and the Military Medical Consortium for the Advancement of Retroviral Research (MMCARR) (1997) Increased drug reaction in HIV-1 positive patients: a possible explanation based on patterns of immune dysregulation seen in HIV-1 disease. Clin Exp Dermatol 22:118–123
105. Wofort FG, Cettrulo CL jr, Nevarre DR (1999) Suction-assisted lipectomy for lipodystrophy syndromes attributed to HIV-protease inhibitor use. Plast Reconstr Surg 104:1814–1820; discussion 1821–1822
106. Vigouroux C, Gharakhanian S, Salhi Y, Nguyen TH, Adda N, Rozenbaum W, Capeau J (1990) Adverse metabolic disorders during highly active antiretroviral treatment (HAART) of HIV disease. Nail and mucocutaneous hyperpigmentation with azidothymidine therapy. J Am Acad Dermatol 22:327–230
107. D'Arminio Monforte A, Testa L, Gianotto M, et al. (1998) Idinavir-related alopecia. AIDS. 12:328
108. Bouscarat F, Bouchard C, Bouhour D (1998) Paronychia and pyogenic granuloma of the great toes in patients treated with Indinavir. N Engl J Med 338:1776–1777
109. Foster RH, Faulds D (1998) Abacavir. Drugs 55:729–736
110. Warner CL, Fiher BK (1986) Cutaneous manifestations of the Acquired Immunodeficiency Syndrome. Int J Dermatol 25:337–349
111. Smith C, Lilly S, Mann KP, Livingston E, Myers S, Lyerly HK, Miralles GD (1998) AIDS-related malignancies. Ann Med 30:323–344

112. Mitsuyasu R (1999) Oncological complications of human immunodeficiency virus disease and hematologic consequences of their treatment. Clin Infect Dis 29:35–43
113. Schulz TF, Boshoff CH, Weiss RA (1996) HIV infection and neoplasia. Lancet 348:587–591
114. Aboulafia DM (1998) Malignant melanoma in an HIV-infected man: a case report and literature review. Cancer Invest 16:217–224
115. Smith C, Lilly S, Mann KP, Livingston E, Myers S, Lyerly HK, Miralles GD (1998) AIDS-related malignancies. Ann Med 30:323–344
116. Ioachim HL, Cooper MC, Hellman GC (1985) Lymphomas in men at high risk for acquired immune deficiency syndrome (AIDS). A study of 21 cases. Cancer 56:2831–2842
117. Bacchi CE, Bacchi MM, Rabenhorst SH, Soares FA, Fonseca LE Jr, Barbosa HS, Weiss LM, Gown AM (1996) AIDS-related lymphoma in Brazil. Histopathology, immunophenotype, and association with Epstein-Barr virus. Am J Clin Pathol 105:230–237
118. Lowenthal D. Straus D, Wise Campbell S, Gold J, Clarkson B, Koziner B (1988) AIDS-related lymphoid neoplasia: the Memorial Hospital experience. Cancer 61:2325–2337
119. Pelicci PG, Knowles DM, Arlin Z, Wieczorek R, et al. (1986) Multiple monoclonal B cell expansions and c-myc oncogene rearrangements in acquired immune deficiency syndrome-related lymphoproliferative disorders. Implications for lymphomagenesis. J Exp Med 164:2049–2076
120. Munoz-Perez MA, Rios-Martin JJ, Rodriguez-Pichardo A, Camacho F (1999) Cutaneous T-cell lymphoma and human immunodeficiency virus infection: 2 cases and a review of the literature. Acta Derm Venereol 79:153–155
121. Dreno B, Milpied HB, Moreau P, Bureau B, Litoux P (1993) Cutaneous anaplastic T-cell lymphoma in a patient with human immunodeficiency virus infection: detection of Epstein-Barr virus DNA. Br J Dermatol 129:77–81
122. Husak R, Mansmann U, Wolfer LU, Geilen CC, Goerdt S, Orfanos CE (1999) Kaposi's sarcoma is an important risk factor for survival in HIV-infected patients independent of $CD4^+$ cell count. AIDS 13:432–433
123. Smith KJ, Nelson A, Angritt P, Morz A, Skelton HG (1999) Kaposi's sarcoma in women: a clinicopathologic study. J Cutan Med Surg 3:132–139
124. Peterman TA, Jaffe HW, Beral B (1991) Epidemiologic clues to the etiology of Kaposi's sarcoma. AIDS 5:135S–142S
125. Brodt HR, Kamps BS, Helm EB, Schofer H, Mitrou P (1998) Kaposi's sarcoma in HIV infection: impact opportunistic infections and survival. AIDS 12:1475–1481
126. Nickoloff BJ, Griffiths CE (1989) The spindle-shaped cells in cutaneous Kaposis's sarcoma. Histologic simulators include factor XIIIa dermal dendrocytes. Am J Pathol 135:793–800
127. Sturzl M, Brandstetter H, Roth WK (1992) Kaposi's sarcoma: a review of gene expression and ultrastructure of KS spindle cells in vivo. AIDS Res Hum Retroviruses 8:1753–1763
128. Browning PJ, Sechler JM, Kaplan M, Washington RH, Gendelman R, Yarchoan R, Ensoli B, Gallo RC (1994) Identification and culture of Kaposi's sarcoma-like spindle cells from the peripheral blood of human immunodeficiency virus-1 in individuals and normal controls. Blood 84:2711–2720
129. Sirianni MC, Uccini S, Angeloni A, Faggioni A, Cottoni F, Ensoli B (1997) Circulating spindle cells: correlation with human herpesvirus (HHV-8) infection and Kaposi's sarcoma Lancet 349:255

Applications of Molecular Virology to Modern Dermatopathology

W. Kempf, D. V. Kazakov, G. Burg

1 Introduction

In the past few decades, molecular virology has led to a dramatic increase in our knowledge of the structure and biology of viruses. For a long time, the identification of infectious organisms had been based on the isolation and cultivation of the pathogen, i.e., growth of the infectious agent in conditioned media or cell cultures, or on the in situ detection in affected tissues, mainly by chromogenic reactions (e.g., Ziehl-Neelsen staining). These methods depend essentially on the replication of pathogens or on the presence of a relatively high number of infectious agents in the affected tissue. Therefore, they are of little use for the detection of infections agents which cannot be cultured, grow poorly, or are present in small numbers in the affected tissue. Molecular biology provided the methodological background for new approaches to the identification of viral components, in particular by employing so-called sequence-based molecular methods (SBMM). SBMM are independent of the replication and isolation of the pathogen. Furthermore, the sensitivity of in vitro nucleic acid amplification techniques allows the detection of very small amounts of viral sequences, even in archival tissue specimens. Thus, SBMM extended dramatically the tools used to search for previously unidentified patho-gens and to detect viral sequences for diagnostic purposes (Relman 1998; Fredricks and Relman 1999).

Many inflammatory and neoplastic skin diseases are considered to be caused by viruses. Recent applications of molecular virology in the search for new viral pathogens have led to the discovery of new pathogens such as human herpesvirus 8 (HHV-8), associated with Kaposi's sarcoma (KS) (Chang et al. 1994). Furthermore, the diagnostic dermatopathological approach to cutaneous viral infections no longer relies exclusively on morphological evaluation but has become extended by new molecular techniques. This chapter reviews the applications of molecular virology to research and diagnosis in modern dermatopathology and highlights some caveats to the interpretation of their results.

Current Topics in Pathology
Volume 94; R. Cerio (Ed.)

2 Sequence-based Molecular Methods

Sequence-based molecular methods are based on the identification of specific DNA or RNA sequences by nucleic acid probes or primers which bind (or hybridize) with a high degree of specificity to complementary DNA or RNA sequences of the pathogen. In the context of general pathology and dermatopathology, the SBMM most widely employed to detect viral pathogens are in situ hybridization (ISH) and the polymerase chain reaction (PCR), including their variants and combinations.

In ISH, the probes target viral nucleic acid sequences which are bound to a solid surface, i.e., a tissue section. The advantage of ISH lies in the ability to localize the hybridization product within the examined specimens and therefore to identify the cell types harboring the infectious agent. Sensitivity is a limiting factor of ISH, since the number of target sequences has to be quite high to be detectable by nucleic acid probes. It has been estimated that about 200 copies of viral sequences have to be present in a single cell of a formalin-fixed, paraffin-embedded tissue section to detect a positive hybridization signal by conventional light microscopy.

The in vitro nucleic acid amplification techniques including PCR, which were developed in the early 1980s, overcome the limitation of low sensitivity by introducing an enzymatic amplification of the nucleic acid sequences of interest. The methodological background and the wide spectrum of PCR applications to dermatopathology have been reviewed elsewhere in detail (Volkenandt et al. 1993; Lo and Feldman 1994; Feldman et al. 1997). Briefly, PCR refers to a process of enzyme-mediated amplification of DNA sequences by repeated cycles of heat denaturation of DNA, annealing of primers to the DNA sequence of interest, and enzyme (= DNA-polymerase)-mediated synthesis of sequence copies (Saiki et al. 1988). After several cycles of amplification, i.e., usually 30–50, billions of copies of the amplified target sequence are generated, which then can be visualized for detection. Thus, even very small amounts of target sequences can be identified in various kinds of specimens. The immense sensitivity and practical applications of PCR render it one of the most widely employed SBMM in general pathology and dermatopathology. Nevertheless, PCR-based methods have their limitations. (a) *Fixation* of tissues or cells with formalin or related substances results in fragmentation of nucleic acids to a length of approximately 400–1200 bp. Nevertheless, PCR can be performed on archival tissue specimens which are decades old, since DNA is relatively resistant to fixation and is very slowly degraded after paraffin embedding (Greer et al. 1991; Mies 1992; Alaibac et al. 1997). The length of amplified products in PCR protocols on archival, i.e., fixed and embedded, tissue is ideally chosen to be smaller than 400–600 bp to avoid false-negative results due to degradation DNA. Since the architecture of investigated tissue is destroyed during DNA or RNA extraction for PCR, the cellular localization of the amplified product is not known. In situ PCR has been developed to combine the sensitivity of PCR and the ability to localize the amplified product in situ (Schiller et al. 1998). (b) *Contamination* is an inherent risk of PCR due to the ability to amplify even smallest amounts of target sequences transferred inadvertently from one to another specimen during preparation and handling of specimens and amplified products. Therefore, strict rules to avoid crossover contamination have to be followed, in particular in the context of diagnostic application of PCR-based methods.

SBMM have been applied to search for known and previously unknown viruses, but also for diagnostic purposes as illustrated in the following.

3 Discovery of Previously Unknown Viruses

Kaposi's sarcoma (KS) is a mesenchymal neoplasm which occurs in four different epidemiological forms (Kempf and Adams 1996). High incidence rates and clustering of KS in certain geographic areas and populations pointed toward a viral pathogen as causative factor. In 1970, CMV was detected in some cases of KS, and during the following two decades several other viruses were supposed as the causative KS viruses (for review see Kempf and Adams 1996). Numerous investigators tried to detect viral components by applying SBMM and other techniques, but none of the proposed viral candidates was consistently found in KS tissue. This led to the hypothesis that a new, not yet known oncogenic virus might be involved in the etiopathogenesis of KS. In 1994, Yuan Chang and Patrick Moore employed a recently developed SBMM, called representational difference analysis (RDA), as an innovative approach to identify the KS virus (Chang et al. 1994). RDA is a method of isolating DNA sequences that are present in one genome, e.g., DNA extracted from tumoral tissue, but absent in another genome such as uninvolved skin, representing the normal counterpart (Lisitsyn 1995). By applying this method, DNA sequences could be identified which were present only in KS tissue (Chang et al. 1994). Sequence analysis revealed that these sequences showed a homology to known herpesviruses such as Epstein-Barr virus. Further investigations confirmed that these viral sequences represented a new, previously unknown herpesvirus called KS-associated herpesvirus, or HHV-8.

Another virus discovered by molecular techniques is the hepatitis C virus (HCV). Screening of a complementary DNA library – constructed from plasma containing an uncharacterized non-A, non-B hepatitis (NANBH) agent – with serum from a patient with NANBH led to the isolation of a unique RNA sequence as part of HCV (Choo et al. 1989). HCV infection is involved in the majority of cases of mixed cryoglobulinemia (MC) and sporadic porphyria cutanea tarda (PCT) (for review see Doutre 1999). Complexes of HCV with IgM/G antibodies have been found in cutaneous vasculitic lesions of MC patients, indicating a direct role of the virus in the pathogenesis of MC (Agnello and Abel 1997). Equivocal data have been reported on the association of HCV with lichen planus (LP), a common inflammatory skin disease. An increased prevalence of serum antibodies against HCV and HCV viremia in a subset of LP patients has been reported (Imhof et al. 1997). Since replication-associated HCV-RNA was not demonstrated in cutaneous LP lesions of patients with chronic hepatitis C, it remains unclear whether HCV is not at all or indirectly involved in the pathogenesis of LP (Mangia et al. 1999). Since lichenoid features can be found in a variety of skin-affecting disorders such as graft-versus-host reactions and drug eruptions, LP probably represents a common pattern of response to various stimuli including viruses.

The etiology of several other inflammatory and neoplastic skin diseases is still unknown, but viruses have been postulated as causative factors. The application of molecular virologic expertise might prove the involvement of already known viruses or result in the discovery of new viruses as the causes of those disorders.

4 Diagnosis and Pathogenetic Aspects of Viral Dermatoses

Not only did molecular virology expand our knowledge about the etiopathogenesis of cutaneous neoplasms, it also resulted in new diagnostic tools and markers. This close relationship between basic research and diagnostic implications of molecular virology is best illustrated by the role of HHV-8 in the diagnosis of KS. Clinically and histologically, KS can mimic various skin diseases, resulting in a broad differential diagnosis (Blumenfeld et al. 1985). Therefore, additional diagnostic markers were needed. As soon as sequences of HHV-8 were discovered, and even before the entire genome was known, the presence of HHV-8 was evaluated as a specific marker for KS. HHV-8 sequences were found in all epidemiological KS forms at a very high prevalence of approximately 95%–100% of KS cases (Ambroziak et al. 1995; Huang et al. 1995), and even in very rare forms such as familial KS (Kempf et al. 1999b). Analysis of numerous vascular and other mesenchymal skin tumors for the presence of HHV-8 revealed HHV-8 DNA sequences to be present only in KS lesions, but not in the other neoplasms examined (Jin et al. 1996; Cathomas et al. 1997). These data indicated that the presence of HHV-8 in mesenchymal neoplasms of the skin can be regarded as a reliable diagnostic marker for KS (Jin et al. 1996).

For the diagnosis of alpha-herpesviruses, i.e., herpes simplex virus (HSV) and varicella-zoster virus (VZV), Nahass and co-workers demonstrated that the detection of HSV and VZV is more sensitive by PCR than using viral culture or cytologic specimens, so-called Tzanck smears (Nahass et al. 1992). In particular, molecular techniques are very helpful in the diagnostic evaluation of cases with atypical manifestation of HSV and VZV infections. Chronic alpha-herpesvirus infections can present with lichenoid or verrucous skin lesions. The characteristic cytolytic changes usually seen in HSV and VZV infections are rarely or not at all detectable in skin biopsies of atypical manifestations by conventional light microscopy. In these cases, the final diagnosis can be established by the detection of viral DNA sequences using PCR and ISH, or by the demonstration of viral antigens using immunohistochemistry (IHC) (Annunziato et al. 1996; Nikkels et al. 1999).

Molecular virologic studies also provided insight into the pathogenesis of cutaneous infections with HSV and VZV. The altered expression of viral proteins may be responsible for a modified or insufficient host immune response, resulting in a chronic course of HSV and VZV infections. In particular, the chronic course of verrucous VZV infections seems to be linked to a particular pattern of VZV gene expression exhibiting reduced synthesis of viral glycoproteins gB and gE (Nikkels et al. 1997). Nikkels and co-workers also demonstrated that the major envelope glycoproteins of HSV and VZV, rather than complete viral particles, might trigger granuloma formation following infection in some cases (Nikkels et al. 1994). In cases of recurrent erythema multiforme (EM), HSV DNA was found in a high percentage of cutaneous lesions, indicating that the prevalence of HSV-related EM is greater than expected, and that PCR might be helpful in identifying patients who could potentially benefit from antiviral therapy (Brice et al.1989).

Human papilloma viruses have been associated with several benign and malignant epithelial tumors (for review see Majewski and Jablonska 1997). Their detection and characterization rely almost exclusively on SBMM. Consensus PCR has been shown to be an efficient approach to detect common HPV sequences shared by numerous HPV types. The most widely used consensus primers bind to the genomic region coding for L1 capsid protein, which shows a high degree of homology within several HPVs. Subsequent amplification with type-specific primers or probes, restriction enzyme digest, and sequence analysis of the amplified products are employed for further HPV typing. In immunocompromised patients such as transplant recipients HPV types can be found which are rarely observed in immunocompetent patients. Using a consensus-PCR protocol and subsequent restriction digest (Adams et al. 1995), we identified HPV type 56 sequence in both verrucae of the hands and perianal condylomata acuminata-like lesions of a renal transplant recipient (Figs. 1, 2) (Kempf et al. 1997). The lesions were ex-

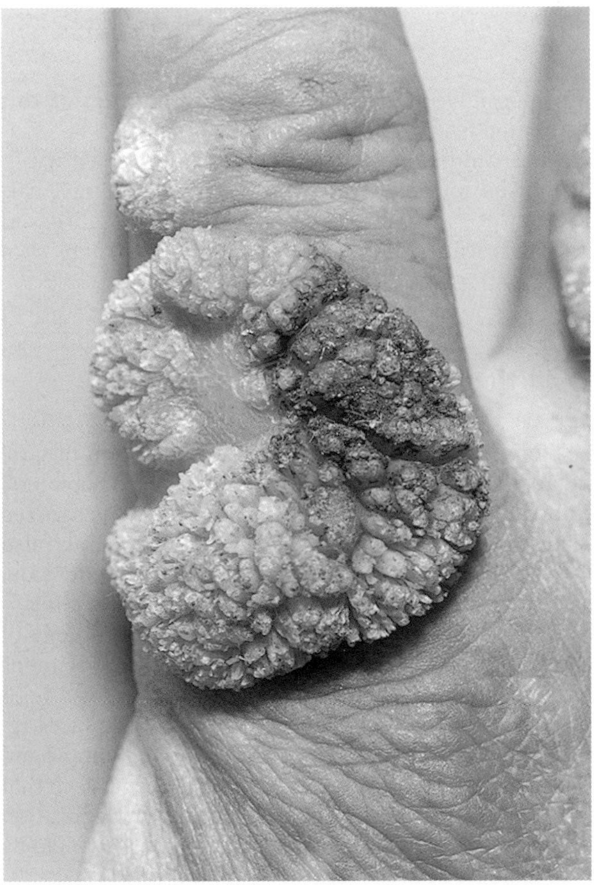

Fig. 1. Giant verrucous lesions on the hand of an immunosuppressed patient after renal transplantation

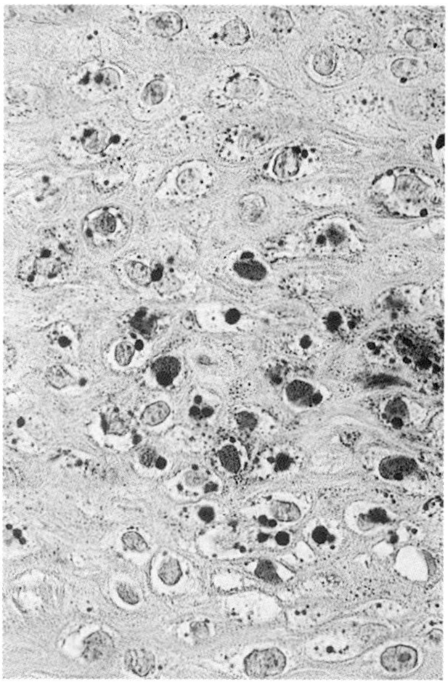

Fig. 2. Immunohistochemical detection of human papilloma virus (HPV) L1 capsid antigen in the lesion (APAAP technique, original magnification ×200), which corresponds to HPV type 56

ceedingly refractory to therapy, possibly owing to the growth properties of this particular HPV type and drug-related immunosuppression.

Interestingly, various HPV types can be detected in the same disease entity. In addition, the same HPV type can be found in various diseases. Therefore, it is difficult to establish an association of particular HPV types to distinct diseases. The prognostic and therapeutic significance of the detection of HPV in many skin diseases remain to be evaluated.

5 Association, Causality, and the Interpretation of Results

SBMM have become relatively simple, very sensitive tools for the detection of viral sequences and have widespread applications. Despite their potential, results obtained using these techniques have to be interpreted very carefully. It is widely recognized that the correct interpretation of skin biopsies by microscopic examination must also take the clinical aspects of the examined lesions into consideration. In extension, molecular virologic findings also have to be interpreted within the context of clinicopathologic features and the biology of the detected virus. Moreover, the biology of many viruses and the significance of the presence of viral sequences in skin specimens are still not entirely clarified and require further studies. It might be simple and obvious, but it must be emphasized that the detection of amplified viral sequences represents primarily only the presence of viral DNA or RNA in the examined sample and does not automatically imply a pathogenetic or even causative role of the virus in that disease. In general, the detection of viral structural proteins indicates viral replication and is a reliable marker of viral infection, whereas the detection of viral sequences by PCR and ISH does not usually distinguish between latent or ongoing infection.

An essential condition for establishing an "association", defined as the reproducibly detectable presence of a pathogen or its components, is consistency of the association. This means that several investigators must be able to detect the pathogen in patients with the disease (reproducibility). There are numerous reports of putative associations between viruses and skin diseases where these postulations have still to be confirmed. Recent examples are contradictory data on the detection of human herpesvirus 7 in pityriasis rosea (Drago et al. 1997; Kempf et al. 1999a) and HHV-8 in sarcoidosis (Di Alberti et al. 1997; Belec et al. 1998; Moore 1998).

The attribution of a causative role of a virus in a disease entity goes far beyond the establishment of an association as described above. Furthermore, the criteria for causality have been changed in the age of molecular biology, and Koch's postulates have been extended and modified (Fredricks and Relman 1996). For example, the discovery of HHV-8 and the subsequent evaluation of its causative role illustrate the broad spectrum of criteria including epidemiological, molecular, and experimental evidence to prove HHV-8 as the causative virus for KS (Moore and Chang 1998).

Virally induced skin diseases, inflammatory and neoplastic ones, represent an attractive topic for research and diagnostic purposes in molecular virology, since the affected tissue is easily accessible via a small biopsy. Nevertheless, the morphological evaluation of skin specimens requires the particular experience of dermatopathologists. For both reasons, dermatopathology plays an essential role in the discovery and detection of viral pathogens.

References

Adams V, Kempf W, Hassam S, Briner J, Schmid M, Moos R, Pfaltz M (1995) Detection of several types of human papilloma viruses in AIDS-associated Kaposi's sarcoma. J Med Virol 46:189–193

Agnello V, Abel G (1997) Localization of hepatitis C virus in cutaneous vasculitic lesions in patients with type II cryoglobulinemia. Arthritis Rheum 40:2007–2015

Alaibac M, Filotico R, Giannella C, Paradiso A, Labriola A, Marzullo F (1997) The effect of fixation type on DNA extracted from paraffin-embedded tissue for PCR studies in dermatopathology. Dermatology 195:105–107

Ambroziak JA, Blackbourn DJ, Herndier BG, Glogau RG, Gullett JH, McDonald AR, Lennette ET, Levy JA (1995) Herpes-like sequences in HIV-infected and -uninfected Kaposi's sarcoma patients. Science 268:582–583

Annunziato P, Lungu O, Gershon A, Silvers DN, LaRussa P, Silverstein SJ (1996) In situ hybridization detection of varicella zoster virus in paraffin-embedded skin biopsy samples. Clin Diagn Virol 7:69–76

Belec L, Mohamed AS, Lechapt-Zalcman E, Authier FJ, Lange F, Gherardi RK (1998) Lack of HHV-8 DNA sequences in sarcoid tissues of French patients. Chest 114:948–949

Blumenfeld W, Egbert BM, Sagebiel RW (1985) Differential diagnosis of Kaposi's sarcoma. Arch Pathol Lab Med 109:123–127

Brice SL, Krzemien D, Weston WL, Huff JC (1989) Detection of herpes simplex virus DNA in cutaneous lesions of erythema multiforme. J Invest Dermatol 93:183–187

Cathomas G, Tamm M, McGandy CE, Itin PH, Gudat F, Thiel G, Mihatsch MJ (1997) Absence of Kaposi's sarcoma-associated human herpes virus 8 in transplantation-related tumors other than Kaposi's sarcoma. Transplant Proc 29:836–837

Chang Y, Cesarman E, Pessin MS, Lee F, Culpepper J, Knowles DM, Moore PS (1994) Identification of herpesvirus-like DNA sequences in AIDS-associated Kaposi's sarcoma. Science 266:1865–1869

Choo QL, Kuo G, Weiner AJ, Overby LR, Bradley DW, Houghton M (1989) Isolation of a cDNA clone derived from a blood-borne non-A, non-B viral hepatitis genome. Science 244: 359–362

Di Alberti L, Piattelli A, Artese L, Favia G, Patel S, Saunders N, Porter SR, Scully CM, Ngui SL, Teo CG (1997) Human herpesvirus 8 variants in sarcoid tissues. Lancet 350:1655–1661

Doutre MS (1999) Hepatitis C virus-related skin diseases. Arch Dermatol 135:1401–1403

Drago F, Ranieri E, Malaguti F, Battifoglio ML, Losi E, Rebora A (1997) Human herpesvirus 7 in patients with pityriasis rosea. Electron microscopy investigations and polymerase chain reaction in mononuclear cells, plasma and skin. Dermatology 195:374–378

Feldman SR, Lye KD, Smith ES, Lo AC, Borcik LD (1997) Polymerase chain reaction and its application for the diagnosis and management of skin diseases. Adv Dermatol 12:115–136

Fredricks DN, Relman DA (1996) Sequence-based identification of microbial pathogens: a reconsideration of Koch's postulates. Clin Microbiol Rev 9:18–33

Fredricks DN, Relman DA (1999) Application of polymerase chain reaction to the diagnosis of infectious diseases. Clin Infect Dis 29:475–488

Greer CE, Peterson SL, Kiviat NB, Manos MM (1991) PCR amplification from paraffin-embedded tissues. Effects of fixative and fixation time. Am J Clin Pathol 95:117–124

Huang YQ, Li JJ, Kaplan MH, Poiesz B, Katabira E, Zhang WC, Feiner D, Friedman-Kien AE (1995) Human herpesvirus-like nucleic acid in various forms of Kaposi's sarcoma. Lancet 345:759–761

Imhof M, Popal H, Lee JH, Zeuzem S, Milbradt R (1997) Prevalence of hepatitis C virus antibodies and evaluation of hepatitis C virus genotypes in patients with lichen planus. Dermatology 195:1–5

Jin YT, Tsai ST, Yan JJ, Hsiao JH, Lee YY, Su IJ (1996) Detection of Kaposi's sarcoma-associated herpesvirus-like DNA sequence in vascular lesions. A reliable diagnostic marker for Kaposi's sarcoma. Am J Clin Pathol 105:360–363

Kempf W, Adams V (1996) Viruses in the pathogenesis of Kaposi's sarcoma – a review. Biochem Mol Med 58:1–12

Kempf W, Adams V, Bachmann P, Schmid M, Mueller B, Burg G (1997) HPV 56 in verrucae of the hands and perianal condylomata acuminata of an immunosuppressed patient with Alport syndrome (abstract). Am J Dermatopathol 19:514

Kempf W, Adams V, Kleinhans M, Burg G, Panizzon RG, Campadelli-Fiume G, Nestle FO (1999a) Pityriasis rosea is not associated with human herpesvirus 7. Arch Dermatol 135:1070–1072

Kempf W, Perniciaro C, Adams V, Mueller B, Burg G (1999b) Human herpesvirus 8 (HHV-8) in familial Kaposi's sarcoma. Exp Dermatol 8:68–70

Lisitsyn NA (1995) Representational difference analysis: finding the differences between genomes. Trends Genet 11:303–307

Lo AC, Feldman SR (1994) Polymerase chain reaction: basic concepts and clinical applications in dermatology. J Am Acad Dermatol 30:250–260

Majewski S, Jablonska S (1997) Human papillomavirus-associated tumors of the skin and mucosa. J Am Acad Dermatol 36:659–685

Mangia A, Andriulli A, Zenarola P, Lomuto M, Cascavilla I, Quadri R, Negro F (1999) Lack of hepatitis C virus replication intermediate RNA in diseased skin tissue of chronic hepatitis C patients. J Med Virol 59:277–280

Mies C (1992) Molecular pathology of paraffin-embedded tissue. Current clinical applications. Diagn Mol Pathol 1:206–211

Moore PS (1998) Human herpesvirus 8 variants. Lancet 351:679–680

Moore PS, Chang Y (1998) Kaposi's sarcoma (KS), KS-associated herpesvirus, and the criteria for causality in the age of molecular biology. Am J Epidemiol 147:217–221

Nahass GT, Goldstein BA, Zhu WY, Serfling U, Penneys NS, Leonardi CL (1992) Comparison of Tzanck smear, viral culture, and DNA diagnostic methods in detection of herpes simplex and varicella-zoster infection. JAMA 268:2541–2544

Nikkels AF, Debrus S, Delvenne P, Sadzot-Delvaux C, Piette J, Rentier B, Pierard GE (1994) Viral glycoproteins in herpesviridae granulomas. Am J Dermatopathol 16:588–592

Nikkels AF, Rentier B, Pierard GE (1997) Chronic varicella-zoster virus skin lesions in patients with human immunodeficiency virus are related to decreased expression of gE and gB. J Infect Dis 176:261–264

Nikkels AF, Snoeck R, Rentier B, Pierard GE (1999) Chronic verrucous varicella zoster virus skin lesions: clinical, histological, molecular and therapeutic aspects. Clin Exp Dermatol 24:346–353

Relman DA (1998) Detection and identification of previously unrecognized microbial pathogens. Emerg Infect Dis 4:382–389

Saiki RK, Gelfand DH, Stoffel S, Scharf SJ, Higuchi R, Horn GT, Mullis KB, Erlich HA (1988) Primer-directed enzymatic amplification of DNA with athermostable DNA polymerase. Science 239:487–491

Schiller PI, Puchta U, Ogilvie AJ, Graf A, Kind P, Sander CA (1998) In situ PCR and PCR in situ hybridization von Paraffin-eingebettetem Gewebe. Neue diagnostische Möglichkeiten in der Pathologie. Pathologe 19:313–317

Volkenandt M, Burmer GC, Schadendorf D, Koch OM, Wienecke R, Degitz K (1993) The polymerase chain reaction. Method and applications in dermatopathology. Am J Dermatopathol 15:118–126

Clinicopathological Differential Diagnosis of Drug-Induced Toxic Epidermal Necrolysis (Lyell's Syndrome) and Acute Graft-Versus-Host Reaction

P. PAQUET, J.E. ARRESE, Y. BEGUIN, G.E. PIÉRARD

1 Introduction

Over the past decades, allogeneic bone marrow transplantation (BMT), also called allogeneic haematopoietic stem cell transplantation (HSCT), has been progressively refined. It evolved from last-resort experiments to first-line therapy for various haematolymphoid malignancies and a few other metabolic disorders. Despite effective immunosuppressive regimens, allogeneic graft-versus-host disease (GVHD) remains a serious and common complication of BMT; mortality increases with GVHD severity [1]. GVHD has also been documented following transplantation of solid organs containing passenger leukocytes. This latter situation is notable for its rarity and its association with high mortality [2]. Contrasting with its deleterious effects, GVHD exhibits an antitumoral effect termed the graft-versus-leukaemia effect. Such a beneficial aspect has also been reported in multiple myeloma and breast cancer.

Autologous and syngeneic GVHD are distinct entities which occur in a minority of patients receiving cyclosporin A after autologous (derived from the recipient) or syngeneic (derived from a monozygotic twin) BMT. They mimic allogeneic GVHD, but generally with milder signs, almost restricted to the skin. It is probably analogous to the eruption of lymphocyte recovery occurring after cytodestructive chemotherapy without BMT.

Current Topics in Pathology
Volume 94; R. Cerio (Ed.)

Nonirradiated blood products contain viable immunological cells capable of inducing GVHD in susceptible hosts. However, transfusion-induced GVHD is infrequent in clinical practice.

Neonatal GVHD has been reported in immunodeficient newborns subsequent to maternal-foetal transfer of immune cells during gestation. The underlying disorders in the neonate are T-lymphocyte deficits, including severe combined immunodeficiency syndrome, Wiskott-Aldrich syndrome and thymic hypoplasia syndromes. The prognosis of neonatal GVHD is grave.

Skin manifestations of GVHD are recognised as two distinct entities: the acute graft versus host reaction (aGVHR), which occurs during the first trimester after BMT, and the chronic type (cGVHR), which includes all the manifestations that develop after the third month following BMT [3]. As a rule, aGVHR is of short duration, involves only the epithelia and is induced by the recognition of host-specific antigens [1]. Cutaneous aGVHR is an early event and a hallmark of GVHD and thus represents an important tool for early diagnosis. Evolving cGVHR consists of relapsing episodes targeting multiple tissues. Its pathobiology remains poorly understood, combining alloimmunity and autoimmunity. Treatment of GVHD varies according to whether the reaction is acute or chronic, making discrimination between types of reaction essential.

A nonspecific pruritic skin rash is often the earliest sign of aGVHR, preceding involvement of the gastrointestinal tract and liver. A morbilliform eruption follows and may progress to severe erythema and blisters. The differential diagnosis of erythematous nonbullous aGVHR includes other complications associated with BMT, including viral exanthem, bacterial and fungal sepsis, cutaneous reaction in response to preparatory regimen (e.g. total body irradiation) and adverse drug reactions. Because therapies of these entities are distinct, it is desirable to render an accurate diagnosis of a post-BMT eruption based on clinical examination in combination with a skin biopsy. When blisters occur after BMT, the main differential diagnosis is drug-induced toxic epidermal necrolysis (TEN), also known under the eponym of Lyell's syndrome.

TEN is a life-threatening disease corresponding to a drug hypersensitivity reaction. The distinction between aGVHR and TEN is a diagnostic and therapeutic challenge, since their treatments are radically different [4–6]. Boosting the immunosuppressive regimen is mandatory in aGVHR, whereas the culprit drug must be discarded without any delay in TEN. Clinical signs are not always sufficient to distinguish between the two disorders [5, 6]. Hence, examination of cutaneous biopsies is commonly performed in order to arrive at the diagnosis. However, morphological and immunohistological aspects of cutaneous aGVHR and those of some drug-induced reactions may look similar. This review compares the clinical presentation and the aetiology, histology and immunohistology of cutaneous aGVHR and TEN, in order to provide potential clues leading to a precise diagnosis.

2 Clinical Features

Cutaneous aGVHR often begins between days 7 and 21 following BMT. A morbilliform or scarlatiniform maculopapular eruption develops and sometimes evolves

Table 1. Clinical cutaneous staging of aGVHR

Stage	Clinical presentation
I	Maculopapular rash involving <25% of body surface
II	Maculopapular rash involving 25%–50% of body surface
III	Generalised erythroderma
IV	Bullous eruption with TEN appearance

to generalised erythroderma. In a minority of cases, blisters develop and remain localised predominantly to pressure sites, but they can spread, with skin flaps sloughing off [1]. Mucosal involvement is poorly documented because it is difficult to distinguish it from chemotherapy-induced mucitis.

Cutaneous aGVHR is classified into four clinical grades, grade IV being the most severe bullous stage (Table 1). It is almost impossible to clinically distinguish grade IV aGVHR from TEN. The time of TEN onset after intake of the culprit drug, the early rash, the subsequent bullous epidermal destruction and the mucous involvement may exhibit morphology and evolution similar to those of aGVHR [4].

Extracutaneous involvement of acute GVHD targets the gastrointestinal tract (diarrhoea, vomiting, abdominal pain, ascites, malabsorption) and/or the liver (increase in levels of aspartate aminotransferase and conjugated bilirubin, jaundice and hepatomegaly). These extracutaneous signs can also be found, although less frequently, in TEN [4].

3 Pathobiology

Acute GVHD occurs when allogeneic immunocompetent cells are introduced into a host unable to reject them. Numerous molecules are responsible for stimulating this alloimmunity. The relative contribution of major and minor histocompatibility (MHC) antigens varies depending on the type of marrow transplant, ranging from related MHC-matched donor and recipient pairs to unrelated and MHC-mismatched pairs or even a xenograft. Some minor transplantation antigens presumably cause GVHD after MHC-matched marrow transplants [7]. The many major and minor antigens are likely to stimulate several effector cell populations, culminating in a mix of lymphocyte types in the epidermis and dermis during aGVHR. Many non-alloreactive lymphocytes are undoubtedly recruited, adding to the heterogeneity. MHC-dependent CD8+ and CD4+ α/β T lymphocytes of donor origin with a highly conserved T-cell receptor repertoire react against host tissue [8]. Donor-derived cytotoxic CD8+ T lymphocytes are responsible in part for the development of aGVHR in allogeneic BMT [9]. In addition, the expression of HLA-DR by keratinocytes allows cytotoxic CD4+ clones to recognise the recipient's peptides presented by class II MHC molecules [10]. In fact, no specific type of lymphocyte can be implicated as a single effector cell of the cutaneous aGVHR [11]. Oligoclonality of T cells mediating aGVHR is established, but not monoclonality [12, 13]. In addition, focusing on just the T lymphocytes neglects contributions to epithelial damage mediated by macrophages and NK cells.

Macrophages and dendrocytes also play a prominent role in aGVHR [14–19]. T lymphocytes, together with the macrophage lineage, are responsible for the production of cytokines, such as IFN-γ and TNF-α, inducing phenotypic changes in keratinocytes, including HLA-DR and adhesion molecule expression [9].

The immunopathology of aGVHR can be conceptualised as three sequential phases resulting from interactions between host tissues, especially epidermal cells, T cells, monocytes and other accessory cells [20]. During the first phase, the conditioning regimen to BMT using irradiation and/or chemotherapy leads to the damage and activation of host tissues, including intestinal mucosa, liver and other tissues, and induces the secretion of the pro-inflammatory cytokines TNF-α and IL-1. As a consequence the expression of both MHC antigens and adhesion molecules is increased, thus enhancing the recognition of host MHC and/or minor histocompatibility antigens by mature donor T cells introduced by allogeneic BMT. During the second phase, donor T-cell activation is characterised by the proliferation of Th-1 cells and the secretion of IL-2 and IFN-γ. Both cytokines induce further T-cell expansion, as well as cytotoxic T-lymphocyte and NK-cell responses, and prime additional mononuclear phagocytes to produce IL-1 and TNF-α. During the third phase, effector functions of mononuclear phagocytes are triggered through secondary signals provided by lipopolysaccharides (LPS) leaking from the damaged intestinal mucosa. LPS subsequently may stimulate gut-associated lymphocytes and macrophages [21]. LPS reaching the skin may also stimulate keratinocytes, fibroblasts and macrophages to produce similar cytokines in the dermis and epidermis. This mechanism results in the amplification of local tissue injury and further promotes an inflammatory response which, together with cytotoxic T lymphocytes and NK cells, leads to target tissue destruction in BMT host.

The main cell types involved in aGVHR (keratinocytes, dendrocytes, macrophages, T lymphocytes) are similarly involved in TEN and other drug reactions [22, 23]. In the TEN initiation phase, the drug metabolite(s) stimulate(s) the keratinocytes to produce TNF-α through a Ca^{++}-related process. In such a process, any increase in the intracellular Ca^{++} influx or mobilisation from the intracellular pool can initiate TNF-α production. In addition, TNF-α promotes the cytosolic Ca^{++} accumulation. TNF-α, acting as an autocrine and paracrine messenger on keratinocytes, stimulates its own production and induces the expression of adhesion molecules and the release of diverse chemotactic factors. The boosted expression of adhesion molecules such as ICAM-1 occurs on keratinocytes in TEN. The monocyte chemotactic protein 1, interleukin-8 (IL-8) and IL-1 are produced by keratinocytes triggered by TNF-α. They act most likely as chemotactic factors for macrophages and T lymphocytes, but this remains unproven in TEN. Based on their location, abutted to the dermal vessels, FXIIIa+ dendrocytes may also participate in the early phase of TEN, acting either as antigen-presenting cells or by attracting inflammatory cells upon secretion of appropriate cytokines.

During the amplification phase, macrophages and T lymphocytes infiltrate the epidermis according to a chemotactic cytokine gradient and cling to cells expressing adequate adhesion molecules. Complex interactions probably exist between these inflammatory cells, leading to the keratinocyte destruction. In fact, activated macrophages produce TNF-α, which is supposedly a major cytokine responsible for the keratinocyte death. The so-called satellite cell necrosis describing T lymphocytes abutted to necrotic keratinocytes is also a key feature linked to the release of perforins [24]. One other mechanism leading to keratinocyte destruction is thought to be apoptosis in both TEN and aGVHR [25–29].

In sum, the many effector cells, the released cytokines, the successive steps in the epidermal destruction and the mode of keratinocyte destruction appear similar in TEN and cutaneous aGVHR. In both diseases, the initial triggering signal is probably localised on the keratinocytes. In TEN, it could result from the toxic action of a drug leading to the recognition of xenobiotic antigens. In aGVHR the recipient's MHC and other molecules serve as unrecognised self-antigens. At least partially common pathogenic mechanisms in both diseases could explain a similar skin involvement.

4 Histological Aspects

Vacuolar alteration of basal cells at the tip of rete ridges and in hair follicles is the earliest evidence of aGVHR which may precede the clinical eruption. In contrast, the skin in a clinically affected area may appear histologically unremarkable [30, 31]. In fact, there is often poor correlation between the clinical aspect of the rash and the microscopic observation.

A histological grading system for aGVHR has been established (Table 2) [30, 32]. However, the basic histopathological parameters, namely, basal vacuolisation, dyskeratotic keratinocytes, subepidermal blistering and epidermal destruction, are not specific for aGVHR.

Nowadays, with modern regimens ablating the haematopoietic and lymphoid systems, the vast majority of aGVHRs show features of grade 1 and 2 disease. Most often there is only a cell-poor superficial lymphocytic infiltrate. When a lichenoid infiltrate is present, it is difficult to distinguish between aGVHR and cGVHR based on examination of skin biopsy specimens alone [33]. Irrespective of the time elapsed after BMT, lichen planus-like features are associated with a two- to sixfold increase in the risk of death from GVHD.

Scattered dyskeratotic keratinocytes, associated or not with abutted lymphocytes, predominate in the deeper epidermis and follicular epithelium. Vasculitis is not typical for aGVHR, although endothelial cell swelling and narrowing of the vascular lumina can be present. Discrete dermal haemorrhage is commonly caused by thrombocytopenia and vascular incompetence. The papillary dermis not infrequently contains a few colloid bodies and scattered melanophages.

Table 2. Histological grading of cutaneous aGVHR

Grade	Microscopical aspect
1	Focal or diffuse vacuolar alteration of basal cells
2	Vacuolar alteration of basal cells, spongiosis and individual apoptotic/necrotic keratinocytes?
3	Subepidermal cleft in association with coalescent necrotic keratinocytes
4	Complete epidermal necrosis and sloughing

Several research groups have tried to fine-tune the histological criteria for a diagnosis of GVHR and have suggested a minimal numerical requirement for dyskeratotic keratinocytes per section length [34], or the requisite presence of a dermal lymphocytic infiltrate [33, 35, 36]. The importance of a lymphoid infiltrate is disputed however, and might not be a prerequisite for the diagnosis of GVHD in any organ [37, 38]. Skin biopsies of low-grade aGVHR do not yield a predictor or a combination of predictors indicating progression to a more severe GVHR [31].

It seems that the skin of severely immunocompromised BMT recipients has only a limited range of reactions. Accordingly, there is significant overlap in the histological appearances of cutaneous eruptions in the post-BMT period.

Several types of drug-induced reactions exhibit similar histological aspects, depending upon when the cutaneous biopsy has been done in the evolution of the disease. In many of these disorders, satellitosis may be present in the epidermis, with lymphocytes engaged in cell-to-cell killing [39]. Polymorphonuclear eosinophils and neutrophils may be present. In contrast, TEN is characterised by a discrete perivascular lymphocytic infiltrate [40]. Only rare cases demonstrate eosinophils or plasma cells. Neutrophils are not encountered [31]. Erythrocyte extravasation in the papillary dermis may be found in some drug-induced reactions and in aGVHR [31]. Eccrine glands are comparably involved in TEN and aGVHR ranging from a moderate degree of epithelial dysplasia to degenerating cells [31, 41]. Hair follicles and sebaceous glands also exhibit altered cells in aGVHR, but this finding is not a feature reported in TEN.

Thus, a skin biopsy is not always useful for differentiating grades I and II aGVHR from other entities that lack specific histological features, such as some drug eruptions and viral exanthems [31, 42]. In other words, the role of skin biopsy is more that of a confirmatory study if other clinical parameters suggest aGVHR and to exclude other processes with specific histological features.

5 Immunohistological Studies

Since histological signs do not provide sufficient clues for discriminating cutaneous aGVHR from some drug-induced dermatitis, several immunohistochemical markers identifying inflammatory cells and adhesion molecules have been proposed to better differentiate these disorders.

5.1 T Lymphocytes

Donor-derived T lymphocytes are the main effector cells responsible for cutaneous lesions of aGVHR. Which T lymphocyte subsets mediate aGVHR is still a matter of controversy, since immunohistological studies do not agree on the composition of the lymphocytic infiltrate. Most authors contend that the skin-infiltrating lymphocytes, in all forms of aGVHR, are memory T cells expressing CD3, CD5, CD45R0 and HLA-DR antigens, with a predominance of CD4+ cells in the dermis and CD8+ in the epidermis [9, 42–49]. Other data are at variance, indicating either equal numbers of CD4+ and CD8+ T lymphocytes in the dermis and epidermis [50, 51], or a predominance of CD4+ T lymphocytes in both tissues [52, 53], or the unique presence of CD8+ in the skin [54].

NK cells may also play a significant role in mediating epidermal cytotoxic damage. Several investigations showed that CD56+ and CD16+ NK cells were present in cutaneous aGVHR [24, 25, 46, 50, 55]. However, some other studies conducted in human subjects did not detect NK cells [47, 50] or identified them in small amounts [9]. Since NK cells lack an epitope-directed receptor, it is likely that they are recruited in a non-specific way by alloantigen-targeted CD4+ and CD8+ lymphocytes [53].

T lymphocytes grossly exhibit the same patterns of distribution in TEN as in aGVHR. A majority of them are present along the dermo-epidermal junction and inside the epidermis. These are CD8+ lymphocytes, whereas the dermal inflammatory infiltrate is composed predominantly of CD4+ cells [56–62]. NK cells are usually rare or absent [56, 57, 59]. Hence, the presence of a number of NK cells might suggest aGVHR rather than TEN.

5.2 Macrophages

The presence of macrophages in aGVHR is rarely reported in the literature [15, 18, 54]. Hence, these cells are not usually considered to play a pivotal role in the disease. However, biopsy specimens from the liver, gut and skin of three patients with lethal GVHD showed a striking preponderance of CD68+ macrophages in the inflammatory infiltrate [15]. Another study showed that monocyte/macrophage L1-protein expression was present in over 80% of aGVHRs [19]. The question about the primary or secondary involvement of macrophages is still open. The macrophage infiltrate observed in some patients might result from a successful anti-lymphocyte effect achieved by steroids and the combined treatments that generally do not target macrophages. However, it cannot be excluded that primary macrophage-mediated aGVHR exists. This situation would logically be unresponsive to causal GVHD treatments targeting specifically lymphocytes.

CD68+ and CD14+ macrophages are present in TEN skin lesions. They have been reported to be less numerous than T lymphocytes [59] or, conversely, more numerous than the latter cells [61, 63–65], especially in the most severely damaged areas of skin. They are located along the dermo-epidermal junction [4, 57] or dispersed in the papillary dermis and epidermis [63, 64].

Macrophages could serve as a clue for the distinction between TEN and aGVHR. When the immunosuppressive regimen to BMT was not efficient enough, the typical aspect of cutaneous aGVHR showed a predominance of T lymphocytes over macrophages. Nowadays, the histological presentation of aGVHR has changed, with refinements in the biological and pharmacological prevention of BMT side effects. The immunosuppressive regimen targets preferentially T lymphocytes, restricting the inflammatory reaction to macrophages [15]. Hence, macrophages are at least as numerous as T lymphocytes in TEN, and even more abundant in most recent cases. Even when macrophages outnumber T lymphocytes in TEN, a pure macrophage infiltrate is never seen. Hence, an inflammatory infiltrate composed almost exclusively of macrophages could be a clue for a lymphocyte-abated aGVHR.

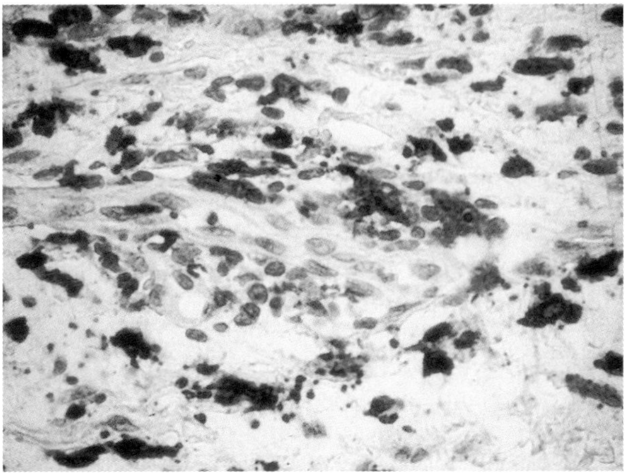

Fig. 1. Numerous plump Factor XIIIa-positive dendrocytes in TEN

5.3 Dendrocytes

CD36+ and Factor XIIIa+ dermal dendrocytes encompass distinct functional subtypes. Their numbers in the superficial dermis are not fixed and have been reported to be increased in the vast majority of TEN cases [19, 62]. The large number of Factor XIIIa+ dendrocytes and their plump appearance in the perilesional and lesional TEN skin (Fig. 1) suggest their activation during the first steps of the disease [62]. Factor XIIIa+ dendrocytes, which are apparently unaffected by the conditioning regimen to BMT [66], appear more numerous and plump in the superficial dermis of most cyclosporine-abated aGVHR [16, 19, 66]. The ultrastructural aspects of these cells are similar in TEN and aGVHR, with dermal dendrocytes showing enlarged endoplasmic reticulum, and phagocytosis of collagen fibres and mast cell granules [16, 19]. It is inferred that both the number and aspect of dermal dendrocytes cannot help in discriminating the two diseases. In contrast, they provide an additional link between them.

5.4 Langerhans' Cells

Epidermal CD1a+, HLA-DR+ Langerhans' cells are remarkably decreased in all grades of cutaneous aGVHR [9, 42, 54, 67, 68]. Langerhans' cell depletion in the epidermis has also been demonstrated in BMT patients who do not develop GVHD, suggesting that it may be due to a toxic effect of a conditioning regimen to BMT [66]. The number of Langerhans' cells is also markedly decreased in TEN epidermis [4, 61, 62]. In TEN, at least two possibilities exist for their depletion. First, they may serve as presenting cells for as yet undefined drug-related antigens and therefore leave the skin to initiate T-cell proliferation. This could be in accordance with the fact that CD1a+ cells are sometimes present in the superficial dermis in TEN [61]. Conversely, Langerhans' cells might be altered, possibly at sites linked with HLA-DR antigens, to become target cells for an autoimmune-type response [56].

5.5 Keratinocytes

Keratinocytes appear to be the main cells in initiating TEN and aGVHR (see Physiopathology). Several immunohistological markers identifying keratinocyte products and adhesion molecules have been proposed to reveal changes in the epidermis of these two conditions.

5.5.1 L1-Protein (Calprotectin)

The 365-kDa L1-protein consists of three calcium noncovalently bound polypeptide chains. It is expressed in neutrophils, monocytes, and some reactive macrophages, as well as in mucosal epithelium and reactive epidermis. Due to its antimicrobial properties, the name calprotectin was coined for it. Keratinocytes underlined by inflammatory cells or covering tumours frequently express the L1-protein, a condition which has been interpreted as a nonspecific marker of cellular stress. The L1-protein persists after formalin fixation and paraffin embedding and is specifically identified using the Mac 387 monoclonal antibody during routine immunohistochemical processing [17] (Fig. 2).

L1-protein keratinocyte expression is present in all cases of cutaneous aGVHR irrespective of the histological grade. The cytoplasmic staining is focal or diffuse all over the epidermal layers, even when the dermal inflammatory infiltrate is scant [17, 38]. The L1-protein keratinocyte expression during aGVHR also probably discloses the sublethal cell injury. Such a finding appears to be very sensitive, although it lacks specificity. An uneven to strong Mac 387+ labelling of keratinocytes is also seen in all biopsies of TEN-altered skin [65] (Fig. 3) The L1-antigen is expressed mainly in suprabasal layers of TEN epidermis, with rare involvement of basal keratinocytes The majority of TEN samples from apparently uninvolved skin express the L1-antigen in a patchy pattern inside the

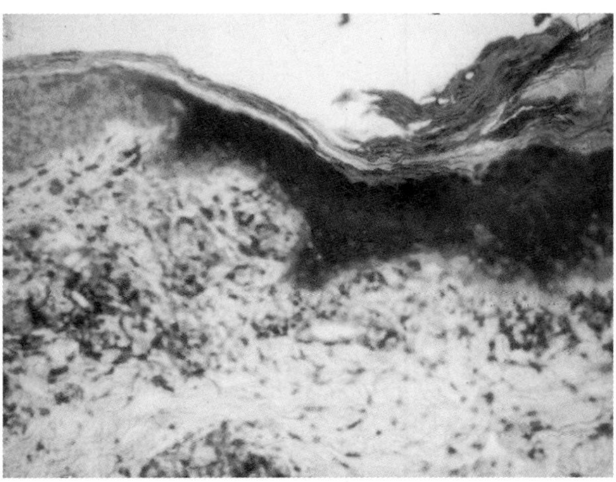

Fig. 2. Mac 387 immunolabelling at the border of an erythematous macule in GVHR. L1-protein-positive monocytes are present in the dermis, and keratinocytes show the expression of calprotectin

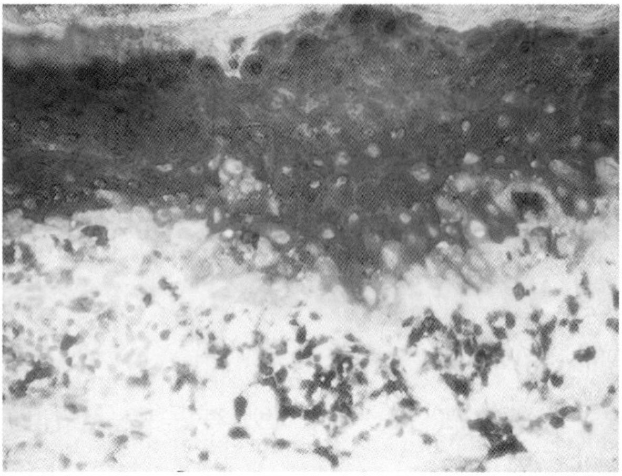

Fig. 3. Mac 387 immunolabelling of keratinocytes and monocytes in the erythematous skin preceding epidermal necrolysis in TEN

epidermis, where inflammatory cells are scant or absent [65]. Hence, epidermal L1-protein expression is not specific and cannot be used to distinguish aGVHR from TEN.

5.5.2 Intercellular Adhesion Molecule-1

Intercellular adhesion molecule-1 (ICAM-1, CD54+) is undetectable on normal keratinocytes. These cells express ICAM-1 throughout the course of aGVHR and even before the lymphocyte infiltration [1, 69]. This expression has been ascribed to the effect of local cytokine (e.g. TNF-α) production and release by infiltrating mononuclear cells [1]. In and around the TEN-damaged keratinocytes, focal areas also stain strongly for ICAM-1 [61].

5.5.3 HLA-DR Expression

HLA-DR molecules are normally absent at the surface of keratinocytes but are found on Langerhans' cells. By contrast, they are also expressed by keratinocytes in the majority of patients with aGVHR [47]. Either HLA-DR displays a focal expression in clumps of basal and suprabasal keratinocytes or it is expressed throughout the entire keratinocyte population [9, 42, 54]. These phenotypic changes have also been considered to be the result of abnormal cytokine stimulation by IFN-γ and TNF-α. The aberrant expression of HLA-DR on keratinocytes is unspecific and has been observed in many inflammatory skin disorders, including TEN [57, 59].

5.5.4 Endothelial Cells

Several studies indicate that modifications of endothelium are involved in aGVHR, probably under the influence of pro-inflammatory cytokines [70]. Vascular adhesion molecules such as E-selectin and vascular-cellular adhesion molecule 1 (VCAM-1) are expressed in aGVHR [71].

In TEN, ICAM-1, ELAM-1 and VCAM-1 are also present on dermal endothelial cells and seem important in the recruitment of the inflammatory cell infiltrate [61]. Hence, there is currently no specific endothelial marker for discriminating TEN and aGVHR.

5.5.5 Miscellaneous Cells

CD45R+ and BA1+ B lymphocytes are rare or absent both in TEN and aGVHR [1, 42, 62]. CD15+ granulocytes are also absent in the two disorders.

6 Conclusion

Definite clinical, histological or immunohistochemical criteria permitting an indisputable distinction between TEN and lymphocyte-depleted aGVHR are not yet available. In fact, a close look at a clinicopathological correlation is required. Consideration must be given to the timing of the biopsy.

Clinically, the main TEN feature that is less often found in aGVHD is the involvement of the mucosae. For example, the ocular signs are almost constant in patients with TEN, but only an estimated 10% of those with severe aGVHD complain of ocular manifestations [72]. The onset of cutaneous symptoms in TEN is also generally more acute and severe than in aGVHR, particularly in the cyclosporine-abated form of the disease. The presence of extracutaneous involvement (liver, gut) can help to support the diagnosis of aGVHD [1].

Conventional histology is of limited usefulness in distinguishing aGVHR from some drug reactions, since all of the diagnostic criteria can at one moment or another be similar in these conditions [4–6, 73]. The density of the inflammatory infiltrate is generally as low in cyclosporine-abated aGVHR as in TEN. Immunohistology can help to reach the diagnosis by increasing the sensitivity in order to detect the epidermal alterations and the nature of the inflammatory cell infiltrate. It may be possible to establish a definite diagnosis of aGVHR through serial skin biopsies and immunohistochemistry in association with close clinicopathological correlation. In such a scenario, the skin biopsy is a tool that can diagnose aGVHR early, before the onset of internal involvement.

References

1. Aractingi S, Chosidow O (1998) Cutaneous graft-versus-host disease. Arch Dermatol 134:602–612
2. Schmuth M, Vogel W, Weinlich G, Margreiter R, Fritsch P, Sepp N (1999) Cutaneous lesions as the presenting sign of acute graft-versus-host disease following liver transplantation. Br J Dermatol 141:901–904
3. Lerner KG, Kao GF, Storb R, Buckner CD, Clift RA, Thomas ED (1974) Histopathology of graft-vs.-host reaction (GvHR) in human recipients of marrow from HLA-matched sibling donors. Transplant Proc 6:367–371
4. Villada G, Roujeau JC, Cordonnier C, Bagot M, Kuentz M, Wechsler J, Vernant JP (1990) Toxic epidermal necrolysis after bone marrow transplantation: study of nine cases. J Am Acad Dermatol 23:870–875
5. McDonald BJ, Singer JW, Bianco JA (1992) Toxic epidermal necrolysis possibly linked to aztreonam in bone marrow transplant patients. Ann Pharmacother 26:34–35
6. Stone N, Sheerin S, Burge S (1999) Toxic epidermal necrolysis and graft vs. host disease: a clinical spectrum but a diagnostic dilemma. Clin Exp Dermatol 24:260–262
7. Wilke M, Poole J, den Hann JM, Goulmy E (1998) Genomic identification of the minor histocompatibility antigen HA-1 locus by allele-specific PCR. Tissue Antigens 52: 303–304
8. Paller AS, Nelson A, Steffan L, Gottschalk L, Kaizer (1988) T-lymphocyte subsets in the lesional skin of allogeneic and autologous bone marrow transplant patients. Arch Dermatol 124:1795–1801
9. Favre A, Amilcare C, Bacigalupo A, Lanino E, Berti E, Grossi C (1987) Immuno-histochemical study of skin lesions in acute and chronic graft-versus-host disease following bone marrow transplantation. Am J Surg Pathol 21:23–24
10. DeBueger M, Bakker A, Van Rood JJ, Goulmy E (1991) Minor histocompatibility antigens, defined by graft-vs.-host disease-derived cytotoxic T lymphocytes show variable expression on human skin cells. Eur J Immunol 21:2839–2344
11. Horn TD, Haskell J (1998) The lymphocytic infiltrate in acute cutaneous allogeneic graft-versus-host reactions lacks evidence for phenotypic restriction in donor-derived cells. J Cutan Pathol 25:210–214
12. Dietrich PY, Caignard A, Lim A, et al. (1994) In vivo T-cell clonal amplification at time of graft-versus-host disease. Blood 84:2815–2820
13. Liu X, Chesnokova V, Forman SJ, Diamond DJ (1996) Molecular analysis of T-cell receptor repertoire in bone marrow transplant recipients: evidence for oligoclonal T-cell expansion in graft-versus-host disease. Blood 87:3032–3044
14. Facon T, Janin A, Noel MP, Jouet JP (1995) Involvement of macrophages in lethal forms of graft-versus-host disease. Lancet 345:392
15. Facon T, Jouet JP, Noel-Walter MP, Bloget F, Bauters F, Janin A (1987) Involvement of TNF-α secreting macrophages in lethal forms of human graft-versus-host disease. Bone Marrow Transplant 20:511–515
16. Yoo YH, Park BS, Whitaker-Menezes D, Korngold R, Murphy G (1998) Dermal dendrocytes participate in the cellular pathology of experimental acute graft-versus-host-disease. J Cut Pathol 25:426–434
17. Piérard GE, Nikkels-Tassoudji N, Arrese J, Nikkels A, Hermanns-Lê T, Piérard-Franchimont C (1998) L1-protein in incipient lymphocyte-depleted graft-versus-host disease. Expression in keratinocytes and co-expression with factor XIIIa in dermal cells. Turk J Dermatopathol 7:10–13
18. Ferrara J, Deeg HJ (1999) Graft-versus-host-disease. N Engl J Med 324:667–374
19. Hermanns-Lê T, Paquet P, Piérard-Franchimont C, Arrese J, Piérard GE (1999) Regulatory function of Factor XIIIa-positive dendrocytes in incipient toxic epidermal necrolysis and graft-versus-host reaction. Dermatology 198:184–186
20. Krenger W, Hill GR, Ferrara J (1987) Cytokine cascades in acute graft-versus-host disease. Transplantation 64:553–558
21. Nestel F, Price K, Seemayer T, Lapp W (1992) Macrophage priming and lipopolysaccharide triggered release of TNF-alpha during graft versus host disease. J Exp Med 175:405–413

22. Barbaud A, Bené MC, Faure G (1987) Immunological physiopathology of cutaneous adverse reactions. Eur J Dermatol 7:319–323
23. Paquet P, Piérard GE (1999) Would cyclosporin A be beneficial to mitigate drug-induced toxic epidermal necrolysis? Dermatology 198:198–202
24. Takata M (1995) Immunohistochemical identification of perforin-positive cytotoxic lymphocytes in graft-versus-host disease. Am J Clin Pathol 103:324–329
25. Gilliam A, Whitaker-Menezes D, Korngold R, Murphy G (1996) Apoptosis is the predominant form of epithelial target cell injury in acute experimental graft versus host disease. J Invest Dermatol 107:377–383
26. Paul C, Wolkenstein P, Adle H, Wechsler J, Garchon HJ, Revuz J, Roujeau JC (1996) Apoptosis as a mechanism of keratinocyte death in toxic epidermal necrolysis. Br J Dermatol 134:710–714
27. Via C, Nguyen P, Shoustov A, Drappa J, Elkon KB (1996) A major role for the Fas pathway in acute graft-versus-host disease. J Immunol 157:5387–5393
28. Yoo YH, Gillian AC, Whitaker-Menezes D, Korngold R, Murphy G (1987) Experimental induction and ultrastructural characterization of apoptosis in murine acute cutaneous graft-versus-host disease. Arch Dermatol Res 289:389–398
29. Viard I, Wehrili P, Bullani R, Schneider P, Holler N, Salomon D, Hunzcker T, Saurat JH, TschoppJ, French LE (1998) Inhibition of toxic epidermal necrolysis by blockade of CD95 with human intravenous immunoglobulin. Sciences 282:490–493
30. Kohler S, Hendrickson MR, Chao NJ, Smoller BR (1987) Value of skin biopsies in assessing prognosis and progression of acute graft-versus-host disease. Am J Surg Pathol 11:988–996
31. Elliot CJ, Sloane JP, Sanderson KV, Vincent M, Shepherd V, Powles R (1987) The histological diagnosis of cutaneous graft versus host disease: relationship of skin changes to marrow purging and other clinical variables. Histopathology 11:145–155
32. Johnson ML, Farmer ER (1998) Graft-versus-host reactions in dermatology. J Am Acad Dermatol 38:369–392
33. Horn TD, Zahurak ML, Atkins E, et al. (1997) Lichen planus-like histopathologic characteristics in the cutaneous graft-vs-host reaction. Prognostic significance independent of time course after allogeneic bone marrow transplantation. Arch Dermatol 133:961–965
34. Horn TD (1994) Acute cutaneous eruptions after marrow ablation: roses by other names? J Cutan Pathol 21:385–392
35. Hymes SR, Farmer ER, Lewis PG, Tutschka PJ, Santos GW (1985) Cutaneous graft-versus-host reaction: prognostic features seen by light microscopy. J Am Acad Dermatol 12: 468–474
36. Sviland L, Pearson AD, Eastham EJ, Hamilton PJ, Proctor SJ, Malcom AJ (1988) Histological features of skin and rectal biopsy specimens after autologous and allogeneic bone marrow transplantation. J Clin Pathol 41:148–154
37. Snover D (1990) The pathology of acute graft-vs-host disease. In: Burakoff SJ (ed) Graft-vs-host disease: immunology, pathophysiology, and treatment. M. Dekker, New York, pp 337–353
38. Piérard GE, Nikkels-Tassoudji N, Nikkels A, Arrese J. Piérard-Franchimont C, Jerusalem G, Beguin Y, Fillet G (1998) Epidermal calprotectin expression in lymphocyte-depleted cutaneous graft-versus-host reaction. Arch Argent Dermatol 48:139–142
39. Saurat JH (1981) Cutaneous manifestations of graft-versus-host disease. Int J Dermatol 20:249–256
40. Paquet P et Piérard GE (1987) Erythema multiforme and toxic epidermal necrolysis. A comparative study. Am J Dermatopathol 19:127–132
41. Akosq AB, Elhag AM (1995) Toxic epidermal necrolysis. A study of the sweat glands. J Cutan Pathol 22:359–364
42. Drijkoningen M, De Wolf-Peeters C, Tricot G, Degreef H, Desmet V (1988) Drug-induced skin reactions and acute cutaneous graft-versus-host reaction: a comparative immunohistochemical study. Blood 56:69–73
43. Sloane J, Thomas J, Imrie S, Easton D, Powlers R (1984) Morphological and immunohistological changes in the skin in allogeneic bone marrow recipients. J Clin Pathol 37:919–930
44. Dreno B, Milpied N, Harousseau J, et al. (1986) Cutaneous immunological studies in the diagnosis of acute graft-versus-host disease. Br J Dermatol 114:7–15

45. Lever R, Turbitt M, Mackie R (1986) A prospective study of the histological changes in the skin in patients receiving bone marrow transplants. Br J Dermatol 114:161–170
46. Elliott C, Sloane J, Pallett C, Sanderson K (1988) Cutaneous leucocyte composition after human allogeneic bone marrow transplantation: relationship to marrow purging, histology and clinical rash. Histopathology 12:1–16
47. Paller S, Nelson A, Steffen L, Gottschalk L, Kaiser H (1988) T-lymphocyte subsets in the lesional skin of allogeneic and autologous bone marrow transplant patients. Arch Dermatol 124:1795–1801
48. Volc-Platzer B, Rappersberger K, Mosberger I, et al. (1988) Sequential immunohistologic analysis of the skin following allogeneic bone marrow transplantation. J Invest Dermatol 91:162–168
49. Girolomoni G, Pincelli C, Zambruno G, et al. (1991) Immunohistochemistry of cutaneous graft-versus-host disease after allogeneic bone marrow transplantation. J Dermatol 18: 314–323
50. Sviland L, Pearson A, Green M, et al. (1991) Immunopathology of early graft-versus-host disease: a prospective study of skin, rectum, and peripheral blood in allogeneic and autologous bone marrow transplant recipients. Transplantation 52:1029–1036
51. Leskinen R, Taskinen E, Volin L, Ruutu T, Häyry P (1992) Immunohistology of skin and rectum biopsies in bone marrow transplant recipients. APMIS 100:1115–1122
52. Takeda H, Mitsuhashi Y, Kondo S, Koto Y, Tajima K (1987) Toxic epidermal necrolysis possibly linked to hyperacute graft-versus-host disease after allogeneic bone marrow transplantation. J Dermatol 24:635–641
53. Horn TD, Haskell J (1998) The lymphocytic infiltrate in acute cutaneous allogeneic graft-versus-host reactions lacks evidence for phenotypic restriction in donor-derived cells. J Cutan Pathol 25:210–214
54. Lampert IA, Janossy G, Suitters A, Bofill M, Palmer S, Gordon-Smith E, Prentice HG, Alero-Thomas J (1982) Immunological analysis of the skin in graft versus host disease. Clin Exp Immunol 50:123–131
55. Acevedo A, Aramburu J, Lopez J, Fernandez-Herrera J, Fernandez-Ranada J, Lopez-Botet M (1991) Identification of natural killer (NK) cells in lesions of human cutaneous graft-versus-host disease: expression of a novel NK-associated surface antigen (Kp43) in mononuclear infiltrates. J Invest Dermatol 97:659–666
56. Merot Y, Gravallese E, Grullen F, Murphy G (1986) Lymphocyte subsets and Langerhans cells in toxic epidermal necrolysis. Arch Dermatol 122:455–458
57. Heng MCY, Allen S (1991) Efficacy of cyclophosphamide in toxic epidermal necrolysis. J Am Acad Dermatol 25:7789786
58. Miyauchi H, Hosokawa H, Akaeda T, Iba H, Asada Y (1991) T-cell subsets in drug-induced toxic epidermal necrolysis. Arch Dermatol 127:851–855
59. Villada G, Roujeau JC, Clerici T, Bourgault I, Revuz J (1992) Immunopathology of toxic epidermal necrolysis. Arch Dermatol 128:50–53
60. Correia O, Delgado L, Ramos J, Resende C, Fleming Torrinha JA (1993) Cutaneous T-cell recruitment in toxic epidermal necrolysis. Arch Dermatol 129:466–468
61. Friedmann P, Strickland E, Permohamed M, Park K (1994) Investigation of mechanisms in toxic epidermal necrolysis induced by carbamazepine. Arch Dermatol 130:598–604
62. Paquet P, Nikkels A, Arrese J, Vanderkelen A, Piérard GE (1994) Macrophages and tumor necrosis factor-α in toxic epidermal necrolysis. Arch Dermatol 130:605–608
63. Friedman HZ, Acias AM, Catchatourian R, Fretzen D (1984) Toxic epidermal necrolysis following bone marrow transplantation. Cutis 34:158–162
64. Roujeau JC, Dubertret L, Moritz D (1985) Involvement of macrophages in toxic epidermal necrolysis. Br J Dermatol 113:425–430
65. Paquet P, Piérard GE (1999) Epidermal calprotectin in drug-induced toxic epidermal necrolysis. J Cutan Pathol 26:301–305
66. Pimpinelli N, Romagnoli A, Alberto B, Santucci M, Mori M, Guidi S Gianotti B (1993) Dendritic cells in the skin after allogeneic bone marrow transplantation: immunohistochemical and electron microscopy monitoring. Eur J Dermatol 3:310–317
67. Murphy GF, Merot Y, Tang ALF (1985) Depletion and repopulation of epidermal dendritic cells after allogeneic bone marrow transplantation in humans. J Invest Dermatol 84: 210–214

68. Perreault C, Pelletier M, Landry D, Gyger M (1995) Study of Langerhans' cells after allogeneic bone marrow transplantation. Blood 63:807–811
69. Norton J, Sloane JP (1991) ICAM-1 expression on epidermal keratinocytes in cutaneous graft-versus-host disease. Transplantation 53:1518–1523
70. Dumler J, Beschorner W, Farmer E, DiGennaro K, Saral R, Santos G (1989) Endothelial cell injury in cutaneous acute graft-versus-host disease. Am J Pathol 135:1097–1103
71. Shen N, French P, Guyotat D (1994) Expression of adhesion molecules in endothelial cells during allogeneic bone marrow transplantation. Eur J Haematol 52:29
72. Jack MK, Jack GM, Sale GE, Schulman HM, Sullivan KM (1983) Ocular manifestations of graft-versus-host disease. Arch Ophthalmol 101:1080–1084
73. Peck GL, Herzig GP, Elios PM (1972) Toxic epidermal necrolysis in a patient with graft-versus-host reaction. Arch Dermatol 105:561–569

Histopathology of Spitz Naevi and "Spitzoid" Melanomas

W.J. Mooi

1 Introduction

The histological distinction between Spitz naevus (Spitz 1948) and a small group of melanomas which resemble Spitz naevus and which are therefore often referred to colloquially as "Spitzoid melanomas" (Smith et al. 1989; Chan et al. 1999) is notoriously difficult and may occasionally be impossible. In the past decades, the recognition of variants of Spitz naevus has resulted in a marked expansion of its clinical and histological spectrum. The differential diagnostic problem is compounded by the fact that like Spitz naevus, Spitzoid melanoma preferentially affects the younger age-groups and may even occur in very young children (Mehregan and Mehregan 1993). In a series of 23 melanomas occurring in children up to 15 years of age, Barnhill (1998) considered three cases to represent Spitzoid melanomas, and a further nine cases were designated "atypical Spitz tumours" (see below), while only six of the cases showed the histology of usual adult-type melanoma. Although there is some evidence to suggest that, as a group, "Spitzoid melanoma" has a more favourable prognosis than other melanomas of similar thickness, there is no doubt that individual examples of Spitzoid melanoma can progress beyond locoregional disease and can kill the patient. A correct diagnosis is therefore of eminent importance. In this brief review, I shall discuss the salient features of Spitz naevi and Spitzoid melanomas, with special emphasis on potential pitfalls and on diagnostically helpful features.

Current Topics in Pathology
Volume 94; R. Cerio (Ed.)

2 Clinical/Macroscopic Features of Spitz Naevus

In the diagnosis of Spitz naevus and of melanoma, clinical features are of central importance and should therefore never be disregarded. Spitz naevi occur predominantly in children, but also in adolescents and young adults, while occasional examples are encountered in late adult life. The face is a favoured site, especially in children, but they may occur anywhere on the skin. Spitz naevi are generally less than 1 cm across, symmetrical, and often raised but only rarely polypoid (Fabrizi and Massi 2000). They are often skin-coloured or reddish but some are pigmented, especially those occurring in adults on the extremities (Dal Pozzo et al. 1997). When pigment is present, it is evenly distributed. A history of recent enlargement or increased pigmentation may be obtained (Crotty et al. 1992). Occasionally, multiple Spitz naevi occur; these may be congenital (Palazzo and Duray 1988) or acquired. Some of these lie grouped together (agminate Hamm et al. 1987) and may arise after removal of a solitary lesion (Sabroe et al. 1996). An association with pregnancy was suggested by a recent case of eruptive Spitz naevi (Onsun et al. 1999).

Very rarely, Spitz naevus has been described in extracutaneous sites, such as the palatal mucosa (Nikai et al. 1990).

Although many cases are not recognised by the clinician as Spitz naevus, clinical suspicion of malignancy is rare. This is an important consideration: A diagnosis of melanoma which comes as a surprise to the clinician should always be discussed between the pathologist and the clinician (Orchard et al. 1997), and the correctness of the diagnosis of melanoma should be critically re-evaluated.

3 Histopathological Features of Spitz Naevus

Only the key features of Spitz naevi will be considered here; for more detailed information, the reader is referred to reviews available elsewhere (Casso et al. 1992; Mooi and Krausz 1992).

3.1 Cytological Features

The single most characteristic histological feature of Spitz naevus is the large size of the pathological melanocytes. These cells often have a large and vesicular nucleus with a prominent nucleolus. As in other naevus types, multinucleated melanocytes may occur, especially in superficial parts. The cytoplasm is usually well-developed, especially superficially, and may have a bluish tinge and ground-glass like appearance. The cells may be rounded or polygonal (epithelioid) or oval to spindle-shaped; the latter are usually somewhat smaller, but still considerably larger than the cells of the common types of melanocytic naevus. Epithelioid cells predominate in Spitz naevi of childhood, whereas spindled melanocytes are more common in lesions of adulthood. Melanin pigment is usually scarce or absent, but it may be abundant in some. When present, the pigment is found superficially and is distributed evenly across the width of the lesion. HMB-45 immunoreactivity is detected in the majority of cases; it is characteristically superficial in location (Bergman et al. 1995a).

3.2 Pathological Architecture

With few exceptions, Spitz naevi are symmetrical, and the histological features vary little from area to area at a given level. Since during its development the naevus spreads regularly in all radial directions, the symmetry is axial, a point that has not always been appreciated in the literature (Okun 1997). As a result, it can be seen histologically regardless of the orientation of individual perpendicular sections. Symmetry should not be taken too literally, however; it means only that eccentric nodules, or markedly asymmetrical and irregular variations in cellularity, cell type, pigmentation, inflammation or fibrosis are absent.

Although, like other naevi, the Spitz naevus probably evolves through a junctional, compound and intradermal phase (Binder et al. 1993), most Spitz naevi are removed when they are compound, involving the epidermis and the dermis. When present, the epidermal component may be sharply demarcated, but this does not need to be the case, so that this feature has little diagnostic applicability (Okun 1998). When there is a junctional component, it is arranged predominantly as nests. When the cells are oval or elongated, nests are usually oval as well and predominantly, but by no means exclusively, vertical in orientation. Some nests are eliminated via the transepidermal route and, in addition, some solitary melanocytes may ascend, especially in the centre of the lesion. This ascent of melanocytes is most common in epithelioid Spitz naevi occurring in young children (Merot and Frenk 1989). In contrast to many ascending melanoma cells, Spitz naevus cells usually diminish in size as they ascend into the upper parts of the epidermis.

There is often reactive epidermal hyperplasia, sometimes to the extent that a designation of pseudoepitheliomatous hyperplasia is appropriate. Especially in the epithelioid variant seen mostly in childhood, the dermal papillae are oedematous and contain ectatic blood vessels (Fig. 1). Clusters of eosinophilic globules, called Kamino bodies (Kamino et al. 1979), may be seen at the dermo-epidermal junction

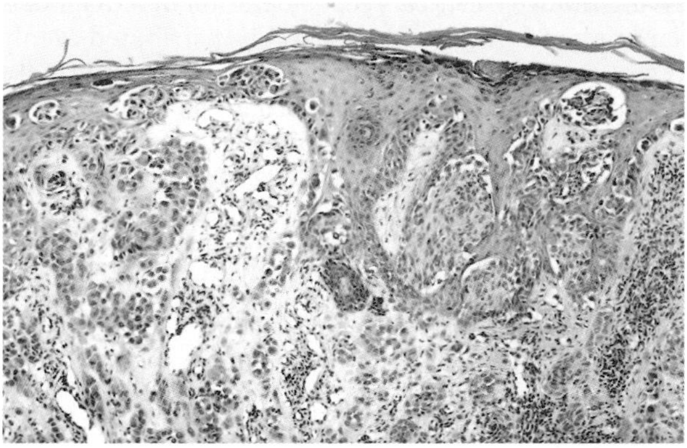

Fig. 1. Spitz naevus, facial skin of a young child. Note the presence of multiple large and small nests of naevus cells in the epidermis and dermis, which is associated with epidermal hyperplasia and dermal oedema and telangiectasia. Ascent of melanocytes into the upper epidermis is not unusual in such epithelioid Spitz naevi

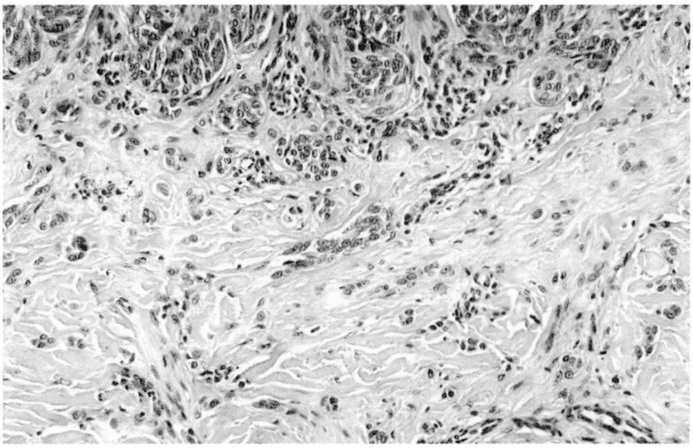

Fig. 2. Deep part of Spitz naevus, showing the characteristic infiltrative rather than compact/ pushing pattern of growth at the base of the lesion. The more richly cellular junctional and subjunctional components of the naevus are just visible at the very top

or in the subepidermal dermis and are diagnostically helpful, since they are rare in melanoma.

The histological features of the base of the Spitz naevus are at least as important as those seen in superficial parts. In the typical example, the pathological melanocytes insinuate themselves singly or in small groups between the collagen fibres of the reticular dermis, without the formation of compact nodules (Fig. 2). The numbers of cells, their size and the size of their nuclei gradually diminish toward the base of the lesion (Bergman et al. 1996). If superficial parts are pigmented, the pigment disappears toward the base. Deep mitotic figures are absent. This disappearance of mitotic activity toward the base is paralleled by a gradual decrease in expression of cyclin D_1 (Nagasaka et al. 1999) and the emergence of deep apoptotic cells (Sprecher et al. 1999). The basal atrophy/"maturation" of the pathological melanocytes is accompanied by loss of expression of the neuronal differentiation marker peripherin, which is present in the superficial part of Spitz naevi (Prieto et al. 1997).

Inflammation is uncommon in Spitz naevi; in particular, groups of plasma cells are rare and their presence should induce a critical reconsideration of a diagnosis of Spitz naevus. When an inflammatory infiltrate is present it is distributed evenly throughout the lesion (Harvell et al. 1997), although it may be slightly more marked at the basal and lateral sides. A clinically apparent halo phenomenon us usually lacking in these Spitz naevi with inflammatory infiltrate.

Generally, Spitz naevus is cured by simple excision; even after incomplete removal, local recurrence is rare, being absent from a series of 49 such cases during a 5-year average follow-up time period (Kaye and Dehner 1990). However, some do recur and may produce multiple lesions, which may be clinically alarming and can compound the histological differential diagnostic difficulties (Sabroe et al. 1996).

4 Main Variants of Spitz Naevus

As indicated above, many variants of Spitz naevus have now been described; these include pigmented (Dellon and Farmer 1988; Dal Pozzo et al. 1997), desmoplastic (Barr et al. 1980), hyalinising (Suster 1994), halo (Yasaka et al. 1995; Harvell et al. 1997), angiomatoid (Diaz-Cascajo et al. 2000), combined (Harvell et al. 1997), plexiform (Spatz et al. 1999b) and pagetoid (Busam and Barnhill 1995) variants. Spitz naevi occasionally occur in combination with other types of melanocytic naevus, such as common acquired naevus (Pulitzer et al. 1991), congenital naevus (Nakagawa et al. 1995) and speckled lentiginous naevus (Aloi et al. 1995).

Most of these variants or combinations are rare or very rare, and space limitations preclude a comprehensive discussion here. However, two less uncommon variants will be briefly considered.

4.1 Desmoplastic Spitz Naevus

Desmoplastic Spitz naevus (Barr et al. 1980) usually presents as a firm, dome-shaped, skin-coloured nodule on an extremity of an adult. Histologically, the lesion is characterised by a usually intradermal proliferation of Spitz-type melanocytes, with characteristic diminution of cell number and cell size toward the base of the lesion and absence of deep mitoses and of compact nodules, accompanied by a characteristic increase in dermal collagen between the pathological melanocytes (Fig. 3). A rare variant of desmoplastic Spitz naevus, characterised by the presence of numerous small blood vessels with plump endothelium within the prominent fibrous naeval stroma, was recently reported by Diaz-Cascajo et al. (2000), under the name of angiomatoid naevus. Desmoplastic Spitz naevus should be distinguished from desmoplastic melanoma, which classically affects

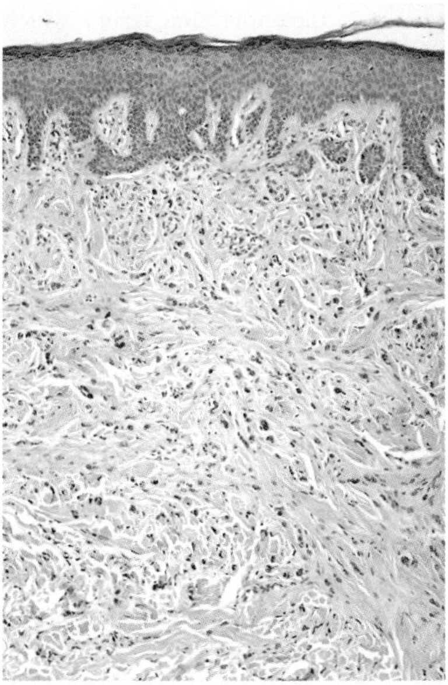

Fig. 3. Desmoplastic Spitz naevus. This largely intradermal proliferation of elongated large melanocytes is accompanied by an increased amount of collagen in a vaguely storiform architecture

the sundamaged skin of elderly patients but may rarely involve covered skin and younger individuals (Chan et al. 1999), and which is characterised histologically by hyperchromatism of long and slender nuclei and by deep mitotic activity.

4.2 Pigmented Spindle Cell Naevus

Pigmented spindle cell naevus (Reed et al. 1975; Barnhill et al. 1991a; Sau et al. 1993) is a small, usually darkly pigmented papule or nodule, most commonly of the skin of the upper leg or thigh region of a young female. The most characteristic histological appearance is a densely cellular proliferation of spindle-shaped melanocytes, forming confluent elongated nests along the dermo-epidermal junction and associated with epidermal hyperplasia, upward spread of pigment within keratinocytes (accounting for the often pitch-black colour), transepidermal elimination of melanocyte nests and also occasional upward spread of solitary melanocytes, usually at the lesion centre (Fig. 4). Kamino bodies may be found at the

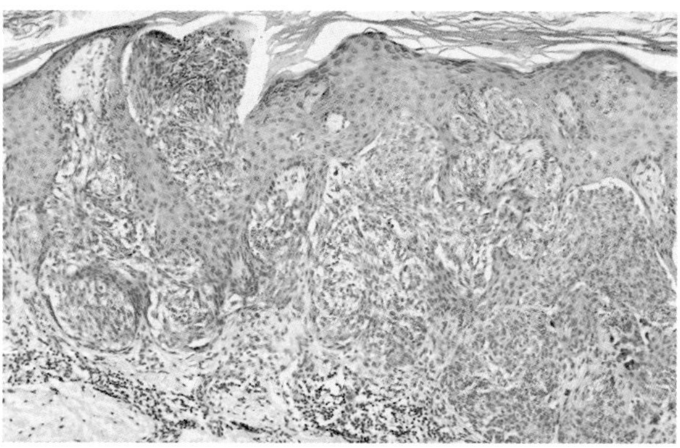

Fig. 4. Pigmented spindle cell naevus. Irregular confluent nests and sheets of elongated melanocytes are flanked and covered by hyperplastic epidermis. There is an inflammatory infiltrate in the underlying dermis, which probably relates to loss of melanin pigment ("pigment incontinence") commonly present in these lesions

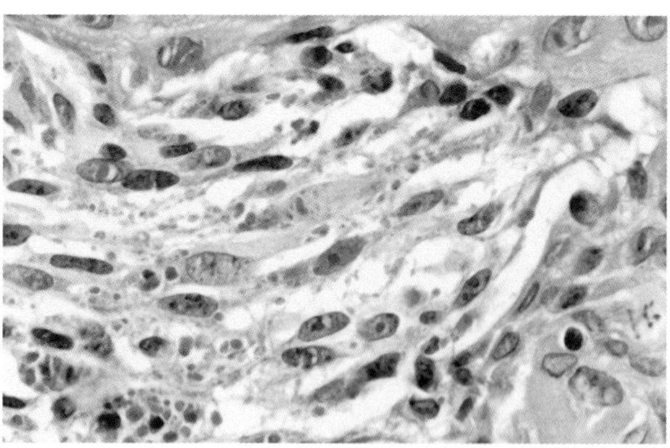

Fig. 5. Pigmented spindle cell naevus. The pathological melanocytes are large, somewhat unequal in appearance, and heavily laden with melanin pigment in this darkly pigmented example. Clinically, such pitch-black nodules may closely resemble pigmented nodular melanoma

junction in the majority of cases (Wistuba and Gonzalez 1990). Loss of pigment into the dermis invokes a moderate inflammatory response in many of these lesions. The pathological melanocytes are usually large, oval to spindle-shaped and often somewhat unequal in appearance, and they may contain large amounts of melanin (Fig. 5). Occasionally, there is overlap with the histology of dysplastic naevus, to the extent that the distinction becomes impossible, and in other cases there may be a combination with areas of common acquired naevus (Barnhill et al. 1991a).

5 Spitzoid Melanoma

Since the spectrum of Spitz naevus is varied, and since the defining feature of Spitzoid melanoma is its histological resemblance to Spitz naevus, it follows that individual Spitzoid melanomas differ considerably from each other. In this brief survey, only the most important and most common features can be outlined.

The tumour cells of Spitzoid melanoma usually exhibit a striking resemblance to Spitz naevus cells. The differential diagnosis cannot usually be made on the basis of cellular detail alone. Architectural features are more important and, significantly, these concern features of not only the upper part of the lesion but also the deep part. Accordingly, a superficial shave biopsy which does not contain the lesion base may prove to be nondiagnostic, while a subsequent excision of the biopsy site may show a heavily traumatised remnant which again may be nondiagnostic. For this reason, an excisional biopsy, which includes the lesion base, is the diagnostic procedure of choice when a skin lesion is suspected to be a Spitz naevus.

The main architectural hallmarks of malignancy which can be found in many Spitzoid melanomas are: filling of the subepidermal region of compact masses or multiple compact nodules of melanocytes; flattening or even thinning of the overlying epidermis (Fig. 6) or, alternatively, exuberant papillomatosis of the epidermis; pagetoid spread of atypical melanocytes also at the edges of the lesion; presence of many mitoses; presence of deep mitoses; presence of atypical mitotic figures; monomorphic cell groups directly adjacent to more pleomorphic cell

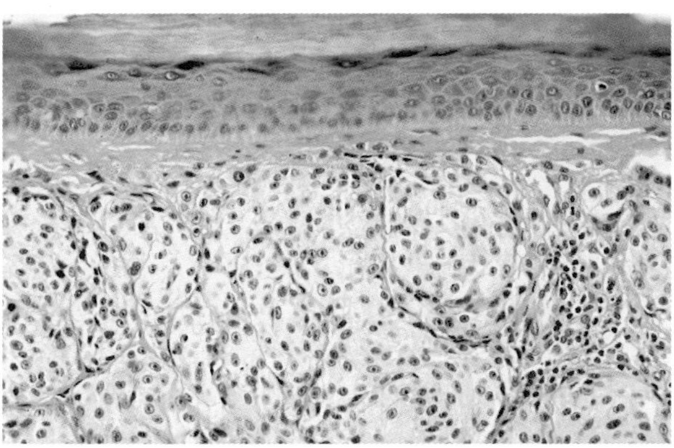

Fig. 6. Spitzoid melanoma. Although the pathological melanocytes resemble Spitz naevus cells, the overlying stretched epidermis, which is devoid of rete ridges, should lead one to question the correctness of a diagnosis of Spitz naevus

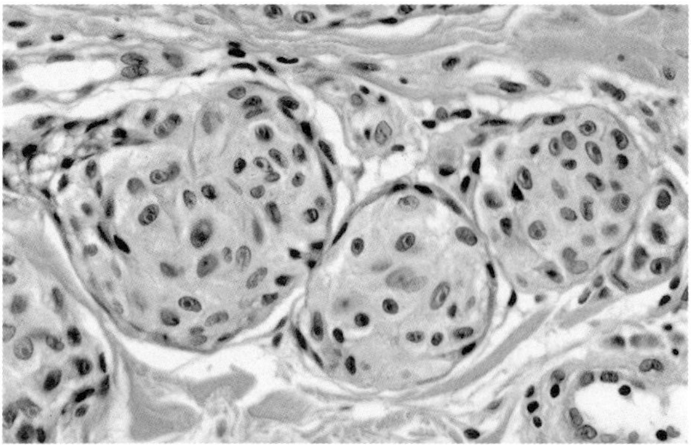

Fig. 7. Spitzoid melanoma, same case as illustrated in Fig. 6. In this deep part of the tumour, the cells still form compact nodules (compare with the characteristic infiltrative pattern of the deep part of Spitz naevus, Fig. 2). This lesion, which occurred on the arm of a young adult, later metastasised to multiple axillary lymph nodes

groups; compact nodules at the base (Fig. 7); irregular distribution of pigment, with nests of melanocytes with dust-like pigment next to amelanotic cell groups. Particularly when these features are found in combination, a diagnosis of Spitzoid melanoma is appropriate. An important additional feature is the variability of cellular features between adjacent cell groups: Cell groups in Spitzoid melanoma vary from each other more than Spitz naevus cell groups do (Fig. 8).

In a recent detailed systematic study of 11 Spitzoid melanomas and 12 Spitz naevi, Walsh et al. (1998) found that the features which best distinguished Spitzoid melanoma from Spitz naevus were: absence of Kamino bodies, brisk mitotic rate, presence of deep mitoses, presence of abnormal mitotic figures, lack of symmetry and lack of uniformity from side to side. From personal experience, I suspect that compact basal architecture, large size of the lesion, and flattening and thinning rather than reactive hyperplasia of the overlying epidermis are of additional diagnostic value. Large size, deep dermal penetration and brisk mitotic activity were also amongst the risk factors identified in the study of Spatz et al. (1999a).

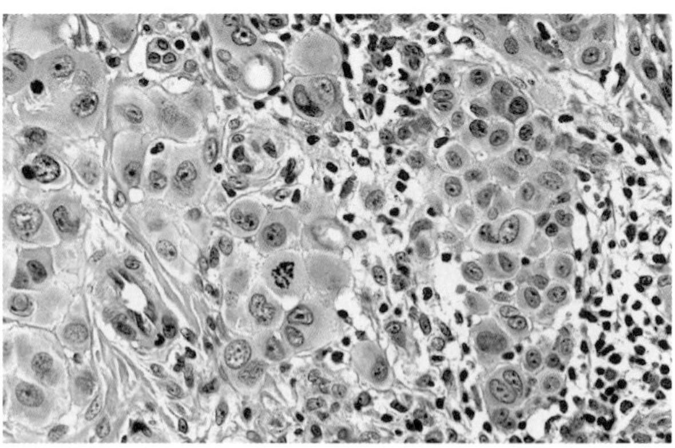

Fig. 8. Spitzoid melanoma, variation in cell type between adjacent cell groups. In Spitzoid melanomas, such abrupt changes in cellular features (cell size, degree of pleomorphism) between adjacent cell groups are often present and aid in the diagnosis

An important diagnostic pitfall is constituted by the so-called deep penetrating naevus (SEAB et al. 1989) and related entities such as the plexiform spindle cell naevus (BARNHILL et al. 1991 b) and some cellular blue naevi and combined naevi. The latter lesions may also exhibit a compact architecture at the base and may show deep pigmentation and some deep mitotic activity. In this respect, it is important to note that some blue naevi are amelanotic, which increases their resemblance to Spitz naevi and Spitzoid melanoma (BHAWAN and CAO 1999). Two cases recently described under the name of "plexiform Spitz naevus" (SPATZ et al. 1999 b) presumably also belong in this category. Finally, some nonmelanocytic skin lesions should be considered in the differential diagnosis. These include cellular neurothekeoma (BARNHILL and MIHM 1990); reticulohistiocytoma (PURVIS and HELWIG 1954) and epithelioid cell histiocytoma (WILSON-JONES et al. 1989).

6 Additional Techniques of Potential Diagnostic Relevance

Various workers have proposed the use of immunohistochemistry and other additional techniques to improve the distinction between Spitz naevus and melanoma. Although the data are in need of independent confirmation, there is reason to hope that some of the parameters put forward will prove to be robust and applicable in a routine diagnostic setting.

In one systematic study, 96% of melanomas but only 6% of Spitz naevi expressed *BCL-2* and had an MIB-1 index exceeding 2% (KANTER-LEWENSOHN et al. 1997). In another study, MIB-1-positive pathological melanocytes in Spitz naevi and melanomas were a mean of 3.2% and 15.3%, respectively (NAGASAKA et al. 1999). The PCNA index (number of PCNA-positive cells per 1000 pathological cells) was significantly lower in Spitz naevus as compared with melanoma (TU et al. 1993). Positivity for p53 protein, as detected with MoAb BP53–12, was more common in primary melanoma than in Spitz naevus, but the difference was not large (35% vs 7%; BERGMAN et al. 1995b). In a recent study, expression of vascular endothelial growth factor was detected in 19 of 45 melanomas but in none of the 17 benign melanocytic melanoma simulators tested, including two Spitz naevi (BAYER-GARNER et al. 1999). These preliminary data are in line with an earlier study demonstrating lower numbers of microvessels in Spitz naevus as compared with melanoma (COCKERELL et al. 1994).

In situ hybridisation with a chromosome-1 centromere probe showed a clear difference in number of aberrant nuclei (with three or more signals per nucleus) per high power field between the 15 Spitz naevi and 15 melanomas tested (DE WIT et al. 1994). In a recent study employing comparative genomic hybridisation (BASTIAN-GARNER et al. 1999), chromosomal aberrations were absent from 13 of 17 Spitz naevi tested; the abnormalities identified in the remaining cases included a gain of 11p and a gain of 7q21-qter; this contrasts with the known frequent abnormalities involving chromosomes 1, 6, 7, 8, 9 and 10 encountered in melanoma. In a subsequent study, WETTENGEL et al. (1999) found numerical abnormalities in only two of 42 Spitz naevi (a gain of chromosome 7 and of 17 in one instance each). DNA aneuploidy is common in melanoma and uncommon in naevi (VOGT et al. 1996); in a recent series, 86% of primary melanomas and 16% of naevi were aneuploid (PILCH et al. 2000).

7 Conclusion

In some instances, however, the diagnosis is practically impossible, and even among experts the discrimination between such "atypical Spitz naevi/tumours" and melanoma is subject to substantial interobserver variation (Barnhill et al. 1999). As a consequence, some workers now use the term "atypical Spitz tumour" for lesions with a close resemblance to Spitz naevus, but with additional worrying features (Barnhill et al. 1995). Although, in my opinion, the use of this term makes a diagnosis out of what is essentially a statement of uncertainty, there is no doubt that there is a group of lesions for which the current histological criteria of Spitz naevus and of melanoma do not allow a confident and unequivocal diagnosis. Further follow-up data will be required in order to refine the distinction between benign and malignant tumours in this problem group. I prefer to state and specify my uncertainty rather than use the term "atypical Spitz tumour", but as long as the clinician understands that the histopathologist is unsure, and therefore that the lesion is potentially malignant, the term "atypical Spitz tumour" can be used. For cases where distinction between Spitz naevus and melanoma is impossible, Spatz and colleagues (1999a) have proposed a grading system for risk stratification, with increased risk associated with age over 10 years, diameter of the lesion exceeding 10 mm, presence of ulceration, involvement of the subcutis, and mitotic activity of at least 6/mm^2.

The term "atypical Spitz *naevus*" should be avoided, since the term naevus is to be used only when the lesion is certainly benign. Designations such as "malignant Spitz naevus" or "metastatic atypical Spitz naevus" (Smith et al. 1989; Nitta et al. 1995; Smith et al. 1998) constitute a contradiction in terms and should not be used: If the lesion metastasises to a lymph node, the diagnosis of Spitzoid melanoma is appropriate. Although the suggestion from an early report (Smith et al. 1989) was that these lesions can metastasise to regional lymph nodes but not beyond, experience from others and myself is that at least some of these tumours can metastasise to distant sites and cause the death of the patient.

Further study of these lesions by means of various additional techniques holds promise for increased diagnostic accuracy in the future. Detailed and precise follow-up data of regional and distant metastasis and of tumour-related death remain the mainstay of definitive classification and of corroboration of diagnostic applicability of any proposed diagnostic parameter.

References

Aloi F, Tomasini C, Pippione M (1995) Agminated Spitz nevi occurring within a congenital speckled lentiginous nevus. Am J Dermatopathol 17:594–598

Barnhill RL (1998) Childhood melanoma. Semin Diagn Pathol 15:189–194

Barnhill RL, Mihm MC jr (1990) Cellular neurothekeoma. A distinctive variant of neurothekeoma mimicking nevomelanocytic tumors. Am J Surg Pathol 14:113–120

Barnhill RL, Barnhill MA, Berwick M, Mihm MC jr (1991a) The histologic spectrum of pigmented spindle cell nevus: a review of 120 cases with emphasis on atypical variants. Hum Pathol 22:52–58

Barnhill RL, Mihm MC jr, Magro CM (1991b) Plexiform spindle cell naevus: a distinctive variant of plexiform melanocytic naevus. Histopathology 18:243–247

Barnhill RL, Flotte TJ, Fleischli M, Perez-Atayde A (1995) Cutaneous melanoma and atypical Spitz tumors in childhood. Cancer 15:1833–1845

Barnhill RL, Argenyi ZB, From L, Glass LF, Maize JC, Mihm MC jr, Rabkin MS, Ronan SG, White WL, Piepkorn M (1999) Atypical Spitz nevi/tumors: lack of consensus for diagnosis, discrimination from melanoma, and prediction of outcome. Hum Pathol 30:513–20

Barr RJ, Morales RV, Graham JH (1980) Desmoplastic nevus. A distinct histologic variant of mixed spindle cell and epithelioid cell nevus. Cancer 46:557–564

Bastian-Garner IB, Hough AJ jr, Smoller BR (1999) Vascular endothelial growth factor expression in malignant melanoma: prognostic versus diagnostic usefulness. Mod Pathol 12:770–774

Bayer-Garner IB, Hough AJ Jr, Smoller BR (1999) Vascular endothelial growth factor expression in malignant melonoma: prognostic and diagnostic usefulness. Mod Pathol 12: 770–774

Bergman R, Dromi R, Tau H, Cohen I, Lichtig C (1995a) The pattern of HMB-45 antibody staining in compound Spitz nevi. Am J Dermatopathol 17:542–546

Bergman R, Shemer A, Levy R, Friedman-Birnbaum R, Trau H, Lichtig C (1995b) Immunohistochemical study of p53 expression in Spitz nevus as compared with other melanocytic lesions. Am J Dermatopathol 17:547–550

Bergman R, Sabo E, Schafer I (1996) Measurement of the maturation parameter by using computer-assisted interactive image analysis may be helpful in the differential diagnosis between compound Spitz nevus and malignant melanoma. Am J Dermatopathol 18:567–570

Bhawan J, Cao SL (1999) Amelanotic blue nevus: a variant of blue nevus. Am J Dermatopathol 21:225–228

Binder SW, Asnong C, Paul E, Cochran AJ (1993) The histology and differential diagnosis of Spitz nevus. Semin Diagn Pathol 10:36–46

Busam KJ, Barnhill RL (1995) Pagetoid Spitz nevus. Intraepidermal Spitz tumor with prominent pagetoid spread. Am J Surg Pathol 19:1061–1067

Casso EM, Grin-Jorgensen CM, Grant-Kels JM (1992) Spitz nevi. J Am Acad Dermatol 27:901–913

Chan GS, Choy C, Ng WK, Chan KW (1999) Desmoplastic malignant melanoma on the buttock of an 18-year-old girl: differentiation from desmoplastic nevus. Am J Dermatopathol 21:170–173

Cockerell CJ, Sonnier G, Kelly L, Patel S (1994) Comparative analysis of neovascularization in primary cutaneous melanoma and Spitz nevus. Am J Dermatopathol 16:9–13

Crotty KA, McCarthy SW, Palmer AA, Ng AB, Thompson JF, Gianoutsos MP, Shaw HM (1992) Malignant melanoma in childhood: a clinicopathologic study of 13 cases and comparison with Spitz nevi. World J Surg 16:179–185

Dal Pozzo V, Benelli C, Restano L, Gianotti R, Cesana BM (1997) Clinical review of 247 case records of Spitz nevus (epithelioid cell and/or spindle cell nevus). Dermatology 194:20–25

Dellon AL, Farmer ER (1988) Pigmented Spitz nevus in an adult. Ann Plast Surg 20:128–132

De Wit PE, Kerstens HM, Poddinghe PJ, Van Muijen GN, Ruiter DJ (1994) DNA in situ hybridization as a diagnostic tool in the discrimination of melanoma and Spitz naevus. J Pathol 173:227–233

Diaz-Cascajo C, Borghi S, Weyers W (2000) Angiomatoid Spitz nevus: a distinct variant of desmoplastic Spitz nevus with prominent vasculature. Am J Dermatopathol 22:135–139

Fabrizi G, Massi G (2000) Polypoid Spitz naevus: the benign counterpart of polypoid malignant melanoma. Br J Dermatol 142:128–132

Hamm H, Happle R, Bröcker E (1987) Multiple agminate Spitz naevi: review of the literature and report of a case with distinctive immunohistochemical features. Br J Dermatol 117:511–522

Harvell JD, Meehan SA, LeBoit PE (1997) Spitz's nevi with halo reaction: a histopathologic study of 17 cases. J Cutan Pathol 24:611–619

Kamino H, Misheloff E, Ackerman AB, Flotte TJ, Greco MA (1979) Eosinophilic globules in Spitz's nevi. New findings and a diagnostic sign. Am J Surg Pathol 1:319–324

Kanter-Lewensohn L, Hedblad MA, Wejde J, Llqarsson O (1997) Immunohistochemical markers for distinguishing Spitz nevi from malignant melanomas. Mod Pathol 10:917–920

Kaye VN, Dehner LP (1990) Spindle and epithelioid cell nevus (Spitz nevus). Natural history following biopsy. Arch Dermatol 126:1581–1583

Mehregan AH, Mehregan DA (1993) Malignant melanoma in childhood. Cancer 15:4096–4103

Merot Y, Frenk E (1989) Spitz nevus (large spindle cell and/or epithelioid cell nevus). Age-related involvement of the suprabasal epidermis. Virchows Arch A Anat Histopathol 415: 97–101

Mooi WJ, Krausz T (1992) Biopsy pathology of melanocytic disorders. Chapman and Hall Medical, London, pp 157–185

Nakagawa S, Kumasaka K, Kato T, Atsumi M, Tagami H (1995) Spitz nevus arising on congenital compound nevus pigmentosus. Int J Dermatol 34:863–864

Nagasaka T, Lai R, Medeiros LJ, Brynes RK, McCourty A, Harada T, Saddik M (1999) Cyclin D1 overexpression in Spitz nevi: an immunohistochemical study. Am J Dermatopathol 21: 115–120

Nikai H, Miyauchi M, Ogawa I, Takata T, Hayashi Y, Okazaki H (1990) Spitz nevus of the palate. Report of a case. Oral Surg Oral Med Oral Pathol 69:603–608

Nitta Y, Ohkochi Y, Hara K (1995) "Malignant Spitz nevus" in a 2-year-old Japanese child. J Dermatol 22:500–503

Okun MR (1997) Sihouette symmetry: an unsupportable histologic criterion for distinguishing Spitz nevi from malignant melanoma. Arch Pathol Lab Med 121:48–53

Okun MR (1998) Histological demarcation of lateral borders: an unsupportable criterion for distinguishing malignant melanoma from Spitz naevus and compound naevus. Histopathology 33:158–162

Onsun N, Saracoglu S, Demirkesen C, Kural YB, Atilganoglu U (1999) Eruptive widespread Spitz nevi: can pregnancy be a stimulating factor? J Am Acad Dermatol 40:866–867

Orchard DC, Dowling JP, Kelly JW (1997) Spitz naevi misdiagnosed histologically as melanoma: prevalence and clinical profile. Australas J Dermatol 38:12–14

Palazzo JP, Duray PH (1988) Congenital agminated Spitz nevi: immunoreactivity with a melanoma-associated antibody. J Cutan Pathol 15: 166–170

Pilch H, Gunzel S, Schaffer U, Tanner B, Heine M (2000) Evaluation of DNA ploidy and degree of DNA abnormality in benign and malignant melanocytic lesions of the skin using video imaging. Cancer 88:1370–1377

Prieto VG, McNutt NS, Lugo J, Reed JA. The intermediate filament peripherin is expressed in cutaneous melanocytic lesions. J Cutan Pathol (1997) 24:145–150

Pulitzer DR, Martin PC, Cohen AP, Reed RJ (1991) Histologic classification of the combined nevus. Analysis of the variable expression of melanocytic nevi. Am J Surg Pathol 15:1111–1122

Purvis WE III, Helwig EB (1954) Reticulohistiocytic granuloma ("reticulohistiocytoma") of the skin. Am J Clin Pathol 24:1005–1015

Reed RJ, Ichinose H, Clark WH, Mihm MC (1975) Common and uncommon melanocytic nevi and borderline melanomas. Sem Oncol 2:119–147

Sabroe RA, Vaingankar NV, Rigby HS, Peachey RD (1996) Agminate Spitz naevi occurring in an adult after the excision of a solitary Spitz naevus: report of a case and review of the literature. Clin Exp Dermatol 21:197–200

Sau P, Graham JH, Helwig EB (1993) Pigmented spindle cell nevus: a clinicopathologic analysis of ninety-five cases. J Am Acad Dermatol 28:565–571

Seab JA, Graham JH, Helwig EB (1989) Deep penetrating nevus. Am J Surg Pathol 13:39–44

Smith KJ, Skelton HG, Lupton GP, Graham JH (1989) Spindle cell and epithelioid cell nevi with atypia and metastasis (malignant Spitz nevus). Am J Surg Pathol 13:931–939

Smith NM, Evans MJ, Pearce A, Wallace WH (1998) Cytogenetics of an atypical Spitz nevus metastatic to a single lymph node. Pediatr Pathol Lab Med 18:115–122

Spatz A, Calonje E, Handfield-Jones S, Barnhill RL (1999a) Spitz tumors in children: a grading system for risk stratification. Arch Dermatol 135:282–285

Spatz A, Peterse S, Fletcher CD, Barnhill RL (1999b) Plexiform Spitz nevus: an intradermal Spitz nevus with plexiform growth pattern. Am J Dermatopathol 21:542–546

Spitz S (1948) Melanomas of childhood. Am J Pathol 24:591–609

Sprecher E, Bergman R, Meilick A, Kerner H, Manov L, Reiter I, Shafer Y, Maor G, Friedman-Birnbaum R (1999) Apoptosis, Fas and Fas-ligand expression in melanocytic tumors. J Cutan Pathol 26:72–77

Suster S (1994) Hyalinizing spindle and epithelioid cell nevus. A study of five cases of a distinctive histologic variant of Spitz's nevus. Am J Dermatopathol 16:593–598

Tu P, Miyauchi S, Miki Y (1993) Proliferative activities in Spitz nevus compared with melanocytic nevus and malignant melanoma using expression of PCNA/cyclin and mitotic rate. Am J Dermatopathol 15:311–314

Vogt T, Stolz W, Glassl A, Abmayr W, Hohenleutner U, Schmoeckel C, Schiffner R, Landthaler M (1996) Multivariate DNA cytometry discriminates between Spitz nevi and malignant melanomas because large polymorphic nuclei in Spitz nevi are not aneuploid. Am J Dermatopathol 18:142–150

Walsh N, Crotty K, Palmer A, McCarthy S (1998) Spitz nevus versus spitzoid malignant melanoma: an evaluation of the current distinguishing histopathologic criteria. Hum Pathol 29:1105–1112

Wettengel GV, Draeger J, Liesewetter F, Schnell H, Neubauer S, Gebhart E (1999) Differentiation between Spitz nevi and malignant melanomas by interphase fluorescence in situ hybridization. Int J Oncol 14:1177–1783

Wilson-Jones E, Cerio R, Smith NP (1989) Epithelioid cell histiocytoma: a new entity. Br J Dermatol 120:185–195

Wistuba I, Gonzalez S (1990) Eosinophilic globules in pigmented spindle cell nevus. Am J Dermatopathol 12:268–271

Yasaka N, Furue M, Tamaki K (1995) Histopathological evaluation of halo phenomenon in Spitz nevus. Am J Dermatopathol 17:484–486

New Concepts in Cutaneous B-Cell Lymphomas

L. Cerroni, H. Kerl

1 Introduction

In the past, studies on malignant lymphomas of the skin focused mostly on mycosis fungoides and other T-cell lymphomas. In recent years, thanks to constant progress being made in immunology and molecular biology, it was recognised that B-cell lymphomas arising primarily in the skin, i.e. primary cutaneous B-cell lymphomas (PCBCLs), represent a distinct and very important group of extranodal lymphomas [1]. They occur far more frequently than is generally believed. The widespread use of immunohistochemical and molecular genetic techniques revealed that many of the cases classified in the past as cutaneous B-cell pseudolymphomas in fact represent low-grade malignant B-cell lymphomas of the skin [2, 3].

It is crucial to distinguish PCBCLs from secondary cutaneous manifestations of extracutaneous (usually nodal) B-cell lymphomas, because treatment strategies are completely different. PCBCL is currently defined as the presence of cutaneous disease alone with no evidence of extracutaneous spread over a period of at least 6 months following complete staging procedures [4, 5].

Many problems still exist concerning the classification of PCBCLs. Some authors maintain that they represent for the most part B-cell lymphomas of germinal centre cell origin, whereas others believe that the majority consists of marginal zone (MALT-like) lymphomas [6–9]. There is also a view that all PCBCLs should be classified as "SALT-type B-cell lymphomas", irrespective of morphological, immunophenotypic, and molecular patterns [10].

PCBCLs must be differentiated from benign (reactive) infiltrates of B lymphocytes within the skin (B-cell pseudolymphomas). Differentiation of benign from malignant cutaneous B-cell infiltrates relies upon evaluation of a constellation of clinical, histopathological, immunophenotypic, and molecular criteria [11]. A list

Current Topics in Pathology
Volume 94; R. Cerio (Ed.)

Table 1. Antibodies useful for the diagnosis of cutaneous lymphoproliferative diseases in routinely-fixed, paraffin-embedded tissue sections[a]

Antibody	CD	Source	Main specificity
271	2	Novocastra	T lymphocytes
PS1	3	Novocastra	Pan-T lymphocytes
I290	4	Novocastra	T-helper lymphocytes
54/B4	5	Novocastra	T lymphocytes, B-CLL
C8/144b	8	Dako	T-suppressor lymphocytes
270	10	Novocastra	CALLA, germinal centre cells
C3D-1	15	Dako	Reed-Sternberg cells, myeloid cells
L26	20	Dako	B lymphocytes
1F8	21	Dako	Dendritic reticulum cells
BerH2	30	Dako	Activated lymphocytes, Reed-Sternberg cells
DF-T1	43	Dako	T lymphocytes, monocytes, myeloid cells
UCHL1	45RO	Dako	T lymphocytes, monocytes, myeloid cells
N-CAM16	56	Novocastra	NK cells
PGM1	68	Dako	Monocytes/macrophages, myeloid cells
mb-1	79a	Dako	B lymphocytes, plasma cells
mic-2	99	Dako	Leucocytes, Ewing's sarcoma
Ig		Dako	Immunoglobulin heavy and light chains
S100		Dako	T-zone histiocytes
MIB1		Dianova	Proliferating cells
8A3		Endogen	β chain of T-cell receptor
124		Dako	bcl-2 protein
PG-B6p		Dako	bcl-6 protein
TdT		Dako	Precursor lymphocytes
TIA-1		Coulter	Cytotoxic lymphocytes
Granzyme-B		Monosan	Cytotoxic lymphocytes
ALK-1		Dako	t(2;5) fusion protein
CS1–4		Dako	EBV-latent membrane protein

[a] All antibodies to be used after antigen retrieval treatment (heat retrieval).

of the most useful antibodies for analysis of cutaneous lymphoproliferative disorders is summarised in Table 1. The most important criteria for diagnosis are clinicopathological correlation and detection of clonality by immunohistology and/or molecular genetic, which can be studied using the polymerase chain reaction (PCR) technique on routinely fixed, paraffin-embedded biopsy specimens. Unfortunately, however, in approximately 30% of cases of PCBCL, neoplastic cells neither express immunoglobulin light chains nor show a monoclonal band by PCR analysis of J_H gene rearrangement.

2 Classification of Cutaneous B-Cell Lymphomas

A classification of PCBCLs has recently been proposed by the European Organization for Research and Treatment of Cancer (EORTC) – Cutaneous Lymphoma Study Group (Table 2) [4]. In the following, we will summarise the most recent developments in some of the entities listed in this classification.

Table 2. EORTC classification of cutaneous lymphomas [4]

T-Cell Lymphomas	B-Cell Lymphomas
Indolent behaviour	Indolent behaviour
Mycosis fungoides	Follicle centre cell lymphoma
Mycosis fungoides with follicular mucinosis	Immunocytoma (marginal zone B-cell lymphoma)
Pagetoid reticulosis	
Large-cell cutaneous T-cell lymphoma, CD30+	
anaplastic	
immunoblastic	
pleomorphic	
Lymphomatoid papulosis	
Aggressive behaviour	Intermediate behaviour
Sézary syndrome	Large B-cell lymphoma of the leg
Large-cell T-cell lymphomas, CD30-	
immunoblastic	
pleomorphic	
Provisional entities[a]	Provisional entities[a]
Granulomatous slack skin	Intravascular large B-cell lymphoma
CTCL, pleomorphic small/medium-sized	Plasmacytoma
Subcutaneous panniculitis-like T-cell lymphoma	

[a] This group includes cutaneous lymphomas with insufficient data to delineate clear-cut clinicopathological entities.

2.1 Cutaneous Follicle Centre Lymphoma

Cutaneous follicle centre lymphoma (FCL) is defined as the neoplastic proliferation of germinal centre cells confined to the skin [12]. The exact incidence of this type of PCBCL is a matter of discussion. Same authors believe that it represents a common type of CBCL [6, 7], whereas others maintain that true FCLs of the skin are very rare [9]. In our opinion, it represents a relatively common subtype of PCBCL.

To this group belong most of the cases named in the past "reticulohistiocytoma of the dorsum" or "Crosti's lymphoma" [13], typically located on the back. The prognosis of patients with cutaneous FCL is favourable. Recurrences are observed in about 50% of the cases, but dissemination to internal organs is rare.

In the majority of cases, histopathology shows a diffuse pattern characterised by the proliferation of centroblasts and centrocytes, admixed with a variable number of immunoblasts, small lymphocytes and histiocytes, and in some cases eosinophils and plasma cells [4]. Sometimes the differentiation from a large B-cell lymphoma can be very difficult [14]. Recent studies showed that a clear-cut follicular pattern can be observed in a distinct proportion of patients [15] (Fig. 1). In fact, in these cases, monoclonality of germinal centres has been proved by immunohistology or by PCR analysis of J_H gene rearrangement after microdissection of germinal centre cells [16, 17]. Many of these cases were probably classified in the past as B-cell follicular pseudolymphoma. Cases of FCL where a few B-cell blasts are admixed with numerous T-lymphocytes have been classified as "T-cell-rich B-cell lymphomas" [18, 19].

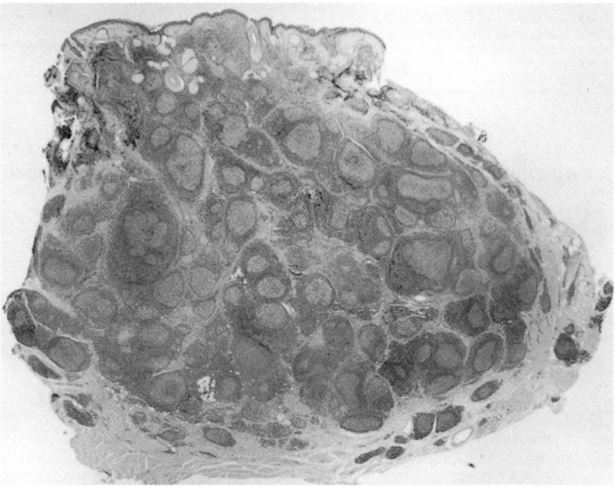

Fig. 1. Cutaneous follicle centre lymphoma, follicular type. Nodular infiltrate of B lymphocytes with prominent follicular pattern

a

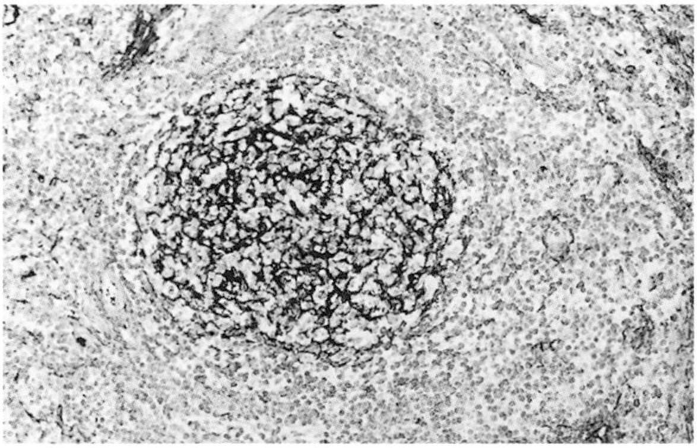

b

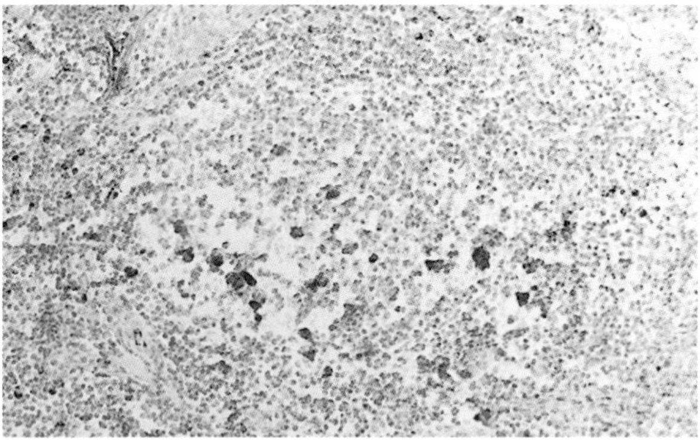

Fig. 2 a, b. Cutaneous follicle centre lymphoma, follicular type. Monoclonality of lymphoid follicles. **a** Positive staining for kappa immunoglobulin light chain; **b** negative staining for lambda immunoglobulin light chain

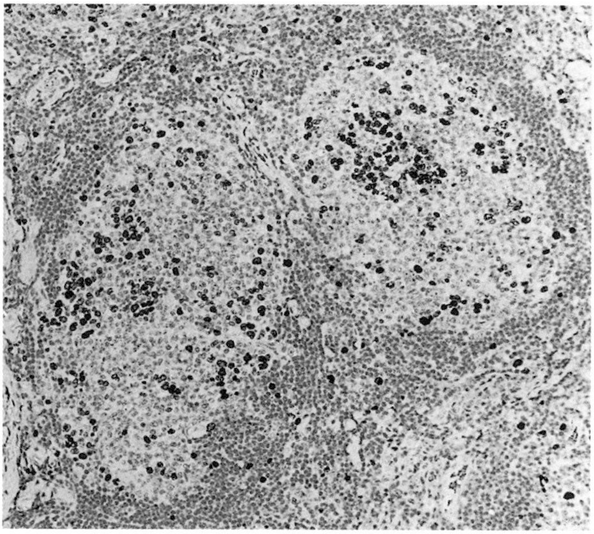

Fig. 3. Cutaneous follicle centre lymphoma, follicular type. Reduced proliferation of lymphoid follicles as detected by the antibody MIB-1

The tumour cells express monotypic surface Ig and B-cell-associated antigens (CD20, CD79a; Fig. 2). Cases characterised by a diffuse growth pattern are CD5, CD10 and CD43 negative, but follicular FCL shows CD10+ cells within neoplastic follicles [17]. Staining for *bcl-2* protein (Bcl-2) yields negative results, which is a major difference from nodal FCL [20]. In about 20% of FCLs of the skin an aberrant positivity for MT2 (CD45RA) can be observed in neoplastic follicles [21]. MT2 positivity is never found within reactive germinal centres and can be considered a useful tool in differentiating cutaneous FCL from B-cell pseudolymphomas. Another useful immunohistochemical feature for differential diagnosis is the lower degree of proliferative activity detected by the MIB-1 antibody in malignant follicles, as opposed to the strong MIB-1 positivity of reactive ones [17] (Fig. 3).

The interchromosomal 14;18 translocation, typically found in nodal follicular lymphomas, is not present in cutaneous FCLs [20, 22]. Analysis of the J_H gene reveals monoclonal rearrangement in the majority of cases.

Synthesis of morphological, immunohistochemical and molecular data suggests that FCLs originating in the lymph nodes and the skin, though characterised by a similar morphological pattern, share different pathogenic mechanisms.

2.2 Cutaneous Marginal Zone Lymphoma

Marginal zone lymphoma (MZL) has recently been recognised as a distinct variant of low-grade malignant PCBCL. It is closely related to immunocytoma and MALT-lymphomas [3, 23]. The prognosis is excellent. In a recent study no patient showed internal involvement after a mean follow-up of more than 4 years [3].

There is lack of agreement among dermatopathologists as to whether MZL and immunocytoma (IC) of the skin represent two distinct entities or should be con-

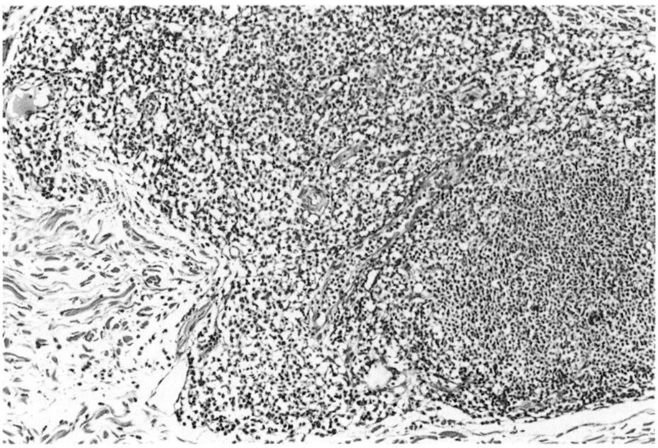

Fig. 4. Cutaneous marginal zone lymphoma. Neoplastic marginal zone cells and plasma cells surround a nodule of small lymphocytes

sidered the two ends of a spectrum of low-grade malignant PCBCL [3, 10, 24–26]. Histology [3] in "classic" cases of MZL shows a characteristic pattern at scanning magnification: nodular infiltrates, sometimes containing reactive germinal centres, are surrounded by a pale-staining population of small to medium-sized cells with indented nuclei, inconspicuous nucleoli and abundant pale cytoplasm (variously described as marginal zone cells, centrocyte-like cells, or monocytoid B-cells) (Fig. 4). In addition, plasma cells (at the margins of the infiltrate), lymphoplasmacytoid cells, small lymphocytes and occasional large blasts are observed (Fig. 5). By contrast, authors considering IC as a separate entity describe an architectural pattern characterised by dense, monomorphous, nodular or diffuse infiltrates with involvement of the dermis and subcutis [3] (Fig. 6). The predominating cell types are lymphoplasmacytoid cells and small lymphocytes (Fig. 7). In addition, plasma cells are usually present, often located at the periphery of the infiltrates. PAS-positive intranuclear inclusions (Dutcher bodies) are sometimes observed and

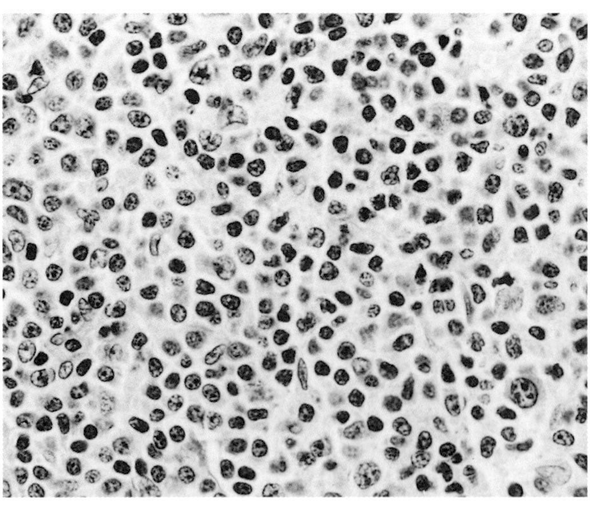

Fig. 5. Cutaneous marginal zone lymphoma. Marginal zone cells with abundant cytoplasm admixed with a few blasts and with lympho-plasmacytoid lymphocytes

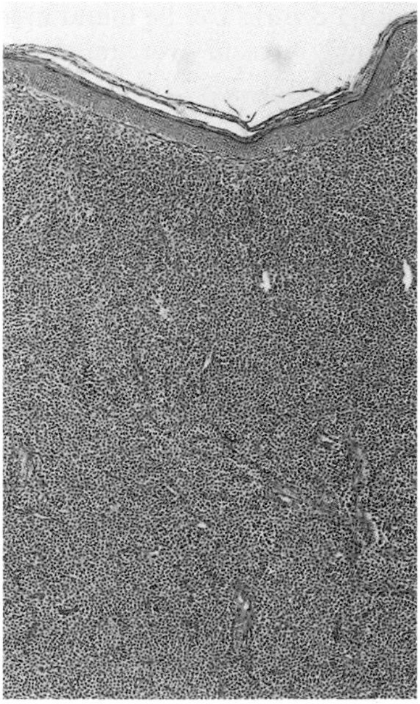

Fig. 6. Cutaneous immunocytoma. Dense infiltrate within the dermis

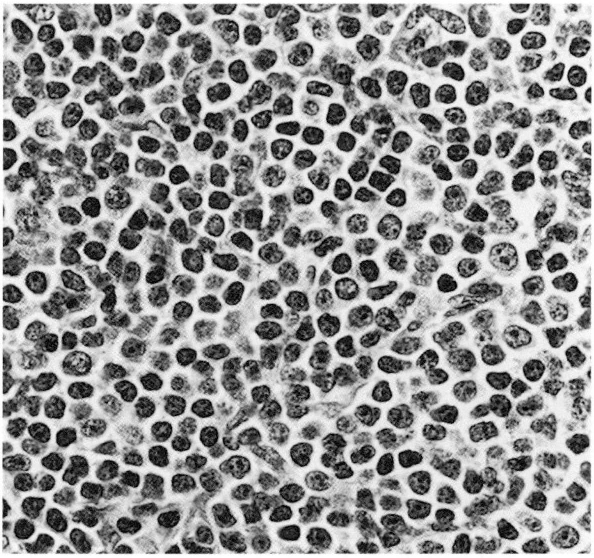

Fig. 7. Cutaneous immunocytoma. Lymphoplasmacytoid lymphocytes predominate within the infiltrate

represent a valuable diagnostic clue. Reactive germinal centres can be found in a few cases. It should be stressed that some patients may present over time with lesions showing histopathological aspects of both MZL and IC.

Neoplastic cells in MZL/IC reveal positivity for CD20, CD79a and Bcl-2, and negativity for CD5 and CD10. In about 65% of cases intracytoplasmic monotypic expression of immunoglobulin light chains can be observed. Staining with the monocytoid B-cell-related antibody Ki-M1p shows a positive reactivity of neoplastic cells with a characteristic intracytoplasmic granular pattern [3]. Monoclonal rearrangement of the J_H genes can be observed in the majority of cases.

2.3 Large B-Cell Lymphoma of the Leg

Large B-cell lymphoma of the leg (LBCL) represents a primary cutaneous B-cell lymphoma characterised by large cell morphology and intermediate prognosis, occurring almost exclusively in elderly, predominantly female, patients. The prognosis is more unfavourable than for other types of PCBCL, with a 5-year survival of approximately 50% [27]. Although the term "large B-cell lymphoma of the leg" is less than optimal, because lesions with similar clinicopathological features can occur also on the skin at sites other than the legs, it refers to the most common location and conveys a peculiar feature of this lymphoma; it parallels other terms accepted in lymphoma pathology such as "hepatosplenic γ/δ T-cell lymphoma" or "nasal lymphoma".

Clinically, patients present with solitary or clustered erythematous or reddish-brown nodules, located mostly on the distal extremity of one leg. Ulceration is

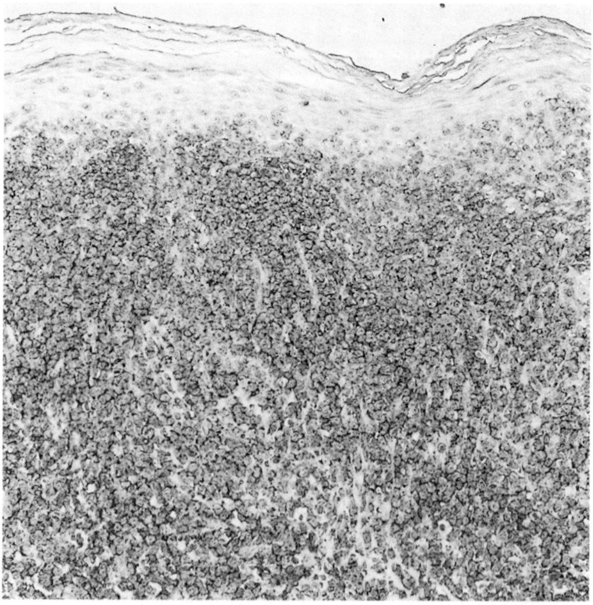

Fig. 8. Cutaneous large B-cell lymphoma. CD20-positive cells within the dermis and involving the epidermis

common. Histology reveals a dense, diffuse infiltrate within the dermis and subcutis [27]. The infiltrate usually involves the entire papillary dermis. Involvement of the epidermis by large neoplastic cells, simulating a T-cell lymphoma, can be observed in rare cases (B-cell epidermotropism) (Fig. 8). The neoplastic infiltrate consists predominantly of immunoblasts and centroblasts. Reactive small lymphocytes are few or absent. Mitoses are frequent. It has been proposed that most cases of LBCL represent large-cell lymphomas originating from lymphocytes of the germinal centre.

Neoplastic cells express monoclonal sIg and/or cIg. B-cell markers and Bcl-2 are positive, but there can be (partial) loss of antigen expression. The tumours reveal monoclonal rearrangement of the J_H genes. The t(14;18) is not present.

2.4 Cutaneous Plasmacytoma

Although in the EORTC classification cutaneous plasmacytoma (PC) is listed only as a provisional entity, a few patients with this type of lymphoma arising primarily in the skin have been described in the literature [28–30]. This type of cutaneous B-cell lymphoma is exceedingly rare. The prognosis is controversial. In fact, although some reports claimed that solitary lesions have a very good prognosis, comparable to that of solitary extramedullary plasmacytoma arising in other tissues, development of multiple myeloma or systemic soft-tissue metastases has been observed in some patients. It seems likely that prognosis in patients with cutaneous PC is related to the tumour burden [30].

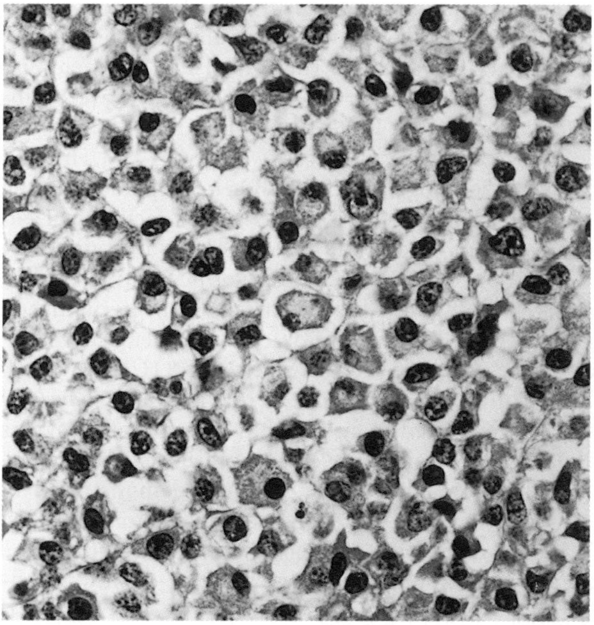

Fig. 9. Cutaneous plasmacytoma. Typical and atypical plasma cells predominate within the infiltrate

The tumour consists of dense nodules and/or sheets of cells within the entire dermis and subcutis [31]. Mature and immature plasma cells with varying degrees of atypia predominate (Fig. 9). Dutcher bodies and Russell bodies are found occasionally. Small, reactive lymphocytes are few or absent. In a few cases amyloid deposits are present within and/or surrounding the neoplastic infiltrates. It should be stressed that presence of amyloid deposition should alert the dermatopathologist to the possibility of extracutaneous PC with skin manifestations. Crystalloid intracytoplasmic inclusions within histiocytes and macrophages may also occur.

Neoplastic plasma cells contain cIg (usually IgA) and show monoclonal expression of one immunoglobulin light chain. CD45 and most B-cell-associated markers are negative, but cells are positive for CD38 in most cases and, less frequently, for CD79a. Immunohistochemical expression of cytokeratins, HMB45 and CD30 can be observed within neoplastic plasma cells, representing a diagnostic pitfall. Molecular analysis usually reveals a monoclonal rearrangement of the J_H genes.

Primary cutaneous plasmacytoma must be differentiated from reactive plasma cell proliferations and from cutaneous inflammatory pseudotumour (plasma cell granuloma) [32]. In reactive conditions plasma cells are not atypical and display a polyclonal pattern of immunoglobulin light chain expression.

3 Identification of Aetiological Agents for Cutaneous B-Cell Lymphoma

In the past, clinical observation of patients with PCBCL revealed that in some cases the lesions were located in close apposition to lesions due to *Borrelia burgdorferi* infection, such as acrodermatitis chronica atrophicans [33]. Recent studies by PCR have revealed that a small percentage (about 20%) of primary cutaneous B-cell lymphomas harbour *B. burgdorferi* DNA sequences within specific skin lesions [34, 35]. *Borrelia*-specific DNA has been observed in all variants of PCBCL, including FCL, MZL/IC and LBCL. It is of interest that, when cases of MZL and IC were subclassified, *Borrelia*-specific DNA was present in 10% of MZLs but in 75% of cases of IC, suggesting a possible difference in aetiology for these two entities [34]. The presence of *B. burgdorferi* underlines the analogies between B-cell lymphomas of the skin and those of the gastric mucosa, where, at least in some cases, infection by *Helicobacter pylori* is considered to be a causative agent [36, 37]. These analogies may also imply that, in at least a small proportion of patients, antibiotic treatment could induce regression of skin lesions. In fact, a few case reports have been published recently showing successful therapy of PCBCL with antibiotic treatment [38, 39].

Other studies investigated the presence of human herpesvirus 8 (HHV-8) DNA within skin lesions of PCBCL. Specific DNA sequences were observed in seven of 63 cases of cutaneous B-cell lymphoma tested so far [40–42]. The role of this virus in the pathogenesis of PCBCL is not yet clear, however. The presence of a functional, constitutively active G-protein-coupled receptor, recently demonstrated in HHV-8, could lead to altered growth and/or neoplastic transformation [43]. Tumour induction by HHV-8 may also follow other pathways related to the presence in the HHV-8 genome of homologues of the cytokine IL-6 and the cell-cycle-control *bcl-2* and cyclin-D genes [44]. However, in view of the recent demonstration of the HHV-8 genome in 5%–10% of the population in certain geographical area, the possibility that HHV-8 positivity in PCBCL represents an epiphenomenon due either to growth of virus in permissive environment or prevalence of it in the general population cannot be excluded with certainty.

4 Conclusions

Very substantial guidelines and criteria for identifying PCBCLs are now available [4, 45, 46]. This has led to the reclassification of several cases that in the past were diagnosed as B-cell pseudolymphomas, and to the identification of various entities with well-defined clinicopathological features. Precise recognition of these entities and identification of aetiological agents will improve the diagnosis and therapy of cutaneous B-cell lymphomas.

References

1. Kerl H, Kresbach H (1979) Lymphoretikuläre Hyperplasien und Neoplasien der Haut. In: Schnyder UW (ed) Spezielle pathologische Anatomie. Springer, Berlin, Heidelberg, New York, pp 396–399
2. Kerl H, Ackerman AB (1993) Inflammatory diseases that simulate lymphomas: cutaneous pseudolymphomas. In: Fitzpatrick TB, Eisen AZ, Wolff K, Freedberg IM, Austen KF (eds) Dermatology in general medicine, 4th edn. McGraw-Hill, New York, pp 1315–1327
3. Cerroni L, Signoretti S, Höfler G, et al. (1997) Primary cutaneous marginal zone B-cell lymphoma. A recently described entity of low-grade malignant cutaneous B-cell lymphoma. Am J Surg Pathol 21:1307–1315
4. Willemze R, Kerl H, Sterry W, et al. (1997) EORTC classification for primary cutaneous lymphomas: a proposal from the Cutaneous Lymphoma Study Group of the European Organization for Research and Treatment of Cancer. Blood 90:354–371
5. Kerl H, Cerroni L (1997) Primary B-cell lymphomas of the skin. Ann Oncol 8 [Suppl 2]: 29–32
6. Willemze R, Rijlaarsdam JU, Beljaards RC, Meijer CJLM (1994) Classification of primary cutaneous lymphomas. Historical overview and perspectives. Dermatology 189:8–15
7. Pimpinelli N, Santucci M, Bosi A, et al. (1989) Primary cutaneous follicular centre-cell lymphoma: a lymphoproliferative disease with favourable prognosis. Clin Exp Dermatol 14:12–19
8. Slater DN (1994) MALT and SALT: the clue to cutaneous B-cell lymphoproliferative disease. Br J Dermatol 131:557–561
9. Isaacson PG, Norton AJ (1994) Cutaneous lymphoma. In: Isaacson PG, Norton AJ (eds) Extranodal lymphomas. Churchill Livingstone, Edinburgh, pp 172–176
10. Santucci M, Pimpinelli N, Arganini L (1991) Primary cutaneous B-cell lymphoma: a unique type of low-grade lymphoma – clinicopathologic and immunologic study of 83 cases. Cancer 67:2311–2326
11. Rijlaarsdam JU, Meijer CJLM, Willemze R (1990) Differentiation between lymphadenosis benigna cutis and primary cutaneous follicular center cell lymphomas: a comparative clinicopathologic study of 57 patients. Cancer 65:2301–2306
12. Kerl H, Kresbach H (1984) Germinal center cell-derived lymphomas of the skin. J Derm Surg Oncol 10:291–295
13. Berti E, Alessi E, Caputo R, Gianotti R, Delia D, Vezzoni P (1988) Reticulohistiocytoma of the dorsum. J Am Acad Dermatol 19:259–272
14. Willemze R, Meijer CJLM, Sentis HJ, et al. (1987) Primary cutaneous large cell lymphomas of follicular center cell origin: a clinical follow-up study of 19 patients. J Am Acad Dermatol 16, 518–526

15. Garcia CF, Weiss LM, Warnke RA, Wood GS (1986) Cutaneous follicular lymphoma. Am J Surg Pathol 10:454–463
16. Cerroni L, Minkus G, Pütz B, Höfler H, Kerl H (1997) Laser dissection of single lymphocytes and PCR analysis in the diagnosis of cutaneous lymphoma. Br J Dermatol 136: 743–746
17. Cerroni L, Arzberger E, Pütz B et al. (2000) Primary cutaneous follicle center cell lymphoma with follicular growth pattern. Blood 95:3922–3928
18. Dommann SN, Dommann-Scherrer CC, Zimmerman D, Dours-Zimmermann MT, Hassam S, Burg G (1995) Primary cutaneous T-cell-rich B-cell lymphoma. A case report with a 13-year follow-up. Am J Dermatopathol 17:618–624
19. Sander CA, Kaudewitz P, Kutzner H, et al. (1996) T-cell-rich B-cell lymphoma presenting in skin. A clinicopathologic analysis of six cases. J Cut Pathol 23:101–108
20. Cerroni L, Volkenandt M, Rieger E, Soyer HP, Kerl H (1994) *bcl-2* Protein expression and correlation with the interchromosomal 14;18 translocation in cutaneous lymphomas and pseudolymphomas. J Invest Dermatol 102:231–235
21. Chimenti S, Cerroni L, Zenahlik P, Peris K, Kerl H (1996) The role of MT2 and anti-bcl-2 protein antibodies in the differentiation of benign from malignant cutaneous infiltrates of B-lymphocytes with germinal center formation. J Cut Pathol 23:319–322
22. Delia D, Borrello MG, Berti E et al. (1989) Clonal immunoglobulin gene rearrangements and normal T-cell receptor, bcl-2, and c-myc genes in primary cutaneous B-cell lymphomas. Cancer Res 49:4901–4905
23. Bailey EM, Ferry JA, Harris NL, Mihm MC jr, Jacobson JO, Duncan LM (1996) Marginal zone lymphoma (low-grade B-cell lymphoma of mucosa-associated lymphoid tissue type) of skin and subcutaneous tissue. A study of 15 patients. Am J Surg Pathol 20: 1011–1023
24. Rijlaarsdam JU, van der Putte SCJ, Berti E, et al. (1993) Cutaneous immunocytomas: a clinicopathologic study of 26 cases. Histopathology 23:117–125
25. Duncan LM, LeBoit PE (1997) Are primary cutaneous immunocytoma and marginal zone lymphoma the same disease? Am J Surg Pathol 21:1368–1372
26. LeBoit PE, McNutt NS, Reed JA, Jacobson M, Weiss LM (1994) Primary cutaneous immunocytoma. A B-cell lymphoma that can easily be mistaken for cutaneous lymphoid hyperplasia. Am J Surg Pathol 18:969–978
27. Vermeer MH, Geelen FAMJ, van Haselen CW, et al. (1996) Primary cutaneous large B-cell lymphomas of the legs. A distinct type of cutaneous B-cell lymphoma with an intermediate prognosis. Arch Dermatol 132:1304–1308
28. Torne R, Su WPD, Winkelmann RK, Smolle J, Kerl H (1990) Clinicopathologic study of cutaneous plasmacytoma. Int J Dermatol 29:562–566
29. Chang YT, Wong CK (1994) Primary cutaneous plasmacytomas. Clin Exp Dermatol 19:177–180
30. Muscardin LM, Pulsoni A, Cerroni L (2000) Primary cutaneous plasmacytoma. Report of a case with review of the literature. J Am Acad Dermatol 43: 962–965
31. Wong KF, Chan JKC, Li LPK, Yau TK, Lee AWM (1994) Primary cutaneous plasmacytoma. Report of two cases and review of the literature. Am J Dermatopathol 16:392–397
32. Hurt MA, Santa Cruz DJ (1990) Cutaneous inflammatory pseudotumor. Am J Surg Pathol 14:764–773
33. Goos M (1971) Acrodermatitis chronica atrophicans and malignant lymphoma. Acta Derm Venereol 51:457–459
34. Cerroni L, Zöchling N, Pütz B, Kerl H (1997) Detection of Borrelia burgdorferi in routinely processed biopsy specimens of primary cutaneous B-cell lymphomas by PCR technique. J Cut Pathol 24:457–461
35. Garbe C, Stein H, Dienemann D, Orfanos CE (1991) Borrelia-burgdorferi-associated cutaneous B-cell lymphoma: clinical and immunohistologic characterization of four cases. J Am Acad Dermatol 24:584–590
36. Wotherspoon AC, Ortiz-Hidalgo C, Falzon MR, et al. (1991) Helicobacter pylori-associated gastritis and primary B-cell gastric lymphoma. Lancet 338:1175–1176
37. Isaacson PG, Spencer J (1993) Is gastric lymphoma an infectious disease? Hum Pathol 24:569–570

38. Kütting B, Bonsmann G, Metze D, Luger TA, Cerroni L (1997) Borrelia burgdorferi-associated primary cutaneous B-cell lymphoma: complete clearing of skin lesions after antibiotic pulse therapy or intralesional injection of interferon alfa-2a. J Am Acad Dermatol 36:311–314
39. Zenahlik P, Fink-Puches R, Kapp KS, Kerl H, Cerroni L (2000) Therapy of primary cutaneous B-cell lymphomas. Hautarzt 51:19–24
40. Sander CA, Simon M, Puchta U, et al. (1996) HHV-8 in lymphoproliferative lesions in skin. Lancet 348:475–476
41. Dupin N, Franck N, Calvez V, et al. (1997) Lack of evidence of human herpesvirus 8 DNA sequences in HIV-negative patients with various lymphoproliferative disorders of the skin. Br J Dermatol 136:827–830
42. Zöchling N, Pütz B, Wolf P, Kerl H, Cerroni L (1998) Human herpesvirus 8-specific DNA sequences in primary cutaneous B-cell lymphomas. Arch Dermatol 134:246–247
43. Arvanitakis L, Geras-Raaka E, Varma A, Gershengorn MC, Cesarman E (1997) Human herpesvirus KSHV encodes a constitutively active G-protein-coupled receptor linked to cell proliferation. Nature 385:347–350
44. Murphy PM (1997) Pirated genes in Kaposi's sarcoma. Nature 385:296–298
45. Kerl H, Cerroni L (1996) The morphologic spectrum of cutaneous B-cell lymphomas. Arch Dermatol 132:1376–1377
46. Cerroni L, Gatter K, Kerl H (1998) An illustrated guide to skin lymphoma. Blackwell Science, Oxford

Clinical and Prognostic Significance of Molecular Studies in Cutaneous T-Cell Lymphoma

S. WHITTAKER

1 Introduction

Mycosis fungoides is the most common form of primary cutaneous T-cell lymphoma (CTCL) and is typically characterised by four cutaneous stages of disease, as described by Bunn and Lamberg [1–3]. In early stages of mycosis fungoides the histological diagnosis can be difficult, and although immunophenotypic studies have helped to distinguish rarer subtypes of primary cutaneous T-cell lymphoma from mycosis fungoides [4], such approaches have not helped in the diagnosis of early-stage disease. While patients with early patch- and plaque-stage disease may have a normal life expectancy, some patients develop tumours or progress to the erythrodermic stages of the disease. Such patients have a median survival of 5 years; the presence of peripheral blood or partial/total lymph node effacement is associated with a poorer prognosis and a median survival of 2.5 years [5]. Significant visceral involvement is usually apparent only in patients who have fulminant disease. Sézary syndrome is characterised by erythroderma, peripheral lymphadenopathy associated with intense pruritus, and the presence of characteristic Sézary cells within peripheral blood. Although most patients with Sézary syndrome have a history of an "eczematous eruption" prior to a diagnosis of cutaneous T-cell lymphoma, some patients with mycosis fungoides gradually develop erythroderma and clinical features indistinguishable from Sézary syndrome. Other independent prognostic factors in mycosis fungoides include age (>60 years) at presentation, which presumably reflects a poorer host immune response in the elderly [6]. Unfortunately, there are no reliable markers of tumour burden in mycosis fungoides. Characteristic Sézary cells may be detected in patients with erythrodermic disease but are rarely present in early-stage disease [7]. Serum IL-2 receptor levels in peripheral blood correlate with prognoses, but only in patients with extensive erythrodermic disease [8]. Similarly, serum LDH levels are elevated only in those patients with significant systemic disease [9]. In contrast, it is known that a small minority of patients with early-stage disease develop progressive cutaneous involvement and systemic disease,

Current Topics in Pathology
Volume 94; R. Cerio (Ed.)

but at present there are no reliable methods for identifying such patients at presentation.

2 Southern Blot Analysis of T-cell Receptor Genes

All lymphocytes undergo somatic rearrangement of either immunoglobulin or T-cell receptor genes. This provides each lymphocyte with a unique rearrangement which produces a diverse immune system and the ability to recognise a wide variety of foreign antigenic peptides. During lymphocyte development, T cells which recognise self-peptides are deleted and those with a productive TCR gene rearrangement can express either an alpha-beta TCR or a gamma-delta TCR. Current evidence suggests that for a minority of peripheral blood T cells the delta gene is rearranged early in T-cell development, followed by the gamma and beta genes. If delta rearrangement is nonproductive, the gene is deleted and alpha rearrangement progresses. While the majority of T cells have a productive rearrangement of either the alpha and beta genes or the gamma and delta genes for a T cell expressing the gamma-delta receptor, a minority will have nonproductive rearrangements and therefore may fail to express a TCR [10]. Southern blot and PCR analysis of both immunoglobulin and TCR genes have been useful methods for identifying clonal lymphoid populations [11–16]. Clonality is synonymous with neoplasia but does not characterise the benign or malignant nature of the tumour. Southern blot and PCR methods are not sensitive enough to detect each individual cell indicated by its unique rearrangement, and so these techniques do not usually identify clonal rearrangements in those patients with antigen-driven lymphoproliferative disorders. Extensive studies in systemic lymphoma have indicated the value of this technique, which now complements traditional pathological and immunophenotypic analysis of systemic nodal lymphomas [11–16]. Southern blot analysis of the beta TCR gene in cutaneous lymphoproliferative disorders has established that a wide variety of conditions have a clonal T-cell origin. These include lymphomatoid papulosis [17, 18], regressing atypical histiocytosis [19], pagetoid reticulosis [20], granulomatous slack skin [21] and follicular mucinosis [22]. In mycosis fungoides T-cell clones can be detected using Southern blot methods in skin biopsies from the majority of patients with late-stage disease but only a small proportion of patients with early plaque stage disease, and usually none with patch-stage disease [23, 24]. Analysis of lymph node material has also shown that TCR gene analysis can provide additional information [23, 25, 26]. Indeed, studies of patients with lymph nodes graded as LN-2 have shown that those with T-cell clones have a worse prognosis than those without [25, 26]. Identical clonal TCR gene rearrangements can be detected in the peripheral blood and skin of patients with later stages of mycosis fungoides, even when peripheral blood films do not show characteristic Sézary cells or expanded $CD4^+$ T-cell populations [24, 27]. However, these Southern blot findings do not appear to have obvious prognostic significance, as peripheral blood T-cell clones are rarely detected using Southern blot methods in patients with early disease.

A variety of V-beta family-specific antibodies are now available commercially and can be used to characterise T-cell populations. Unfortunately, these antibodies do not cover all the known V-beta families and individual antibodies may not identify all the gene segments expressed by T cells utilising a specific V-beta family. However, these antibodies can provide a useful clonotypic marker in patients with either Sézary syndrome or mycosis fungoides. In some cases of mycosis fungoides, studies have indicated that the epidermotropic cells are composed predominantly of T cells expressing a single V-beta gene family [28]. However molecular analysis has suggested that not all these T cells represent the clonal population [29]. Similarly, abnormal phenotypic expression of various lymphoid differentiation markers does not always reliably identify a tumour population. While some patients with Sézary syndrome have T cells with a $CD4^+$, $CD7^-$ phenotype, it is clear that the reverse can also occur, and some patients with mycosis fungoides have $CD8^+$ tumour cells [30, 31].

Therefore, within the limits of its sensitivity, Southern blot analysis of TCR genes has proved to be a very helpful diagnostic aid to conventional pathology and immunophenotypic studies in mycosis fungoides, and analysis of lymph node material may provide additional prognostic information.

3 PCR Analysis of T-Cell Receptor Genes

The use of PCR amplification of T-cell receptor and immunoglobulin genes has improved the detection sensitivity for the identification of clonal rearrangements in fresh or frozen material [15, 16]. In some situations DNA extracted from formalin-fixed, paraffin-embedded material can also be successfully amplified, although DNA degradation due to prolonged formaldehyde exposure and the presence of inhibitors of taq polymerase can prevent successful amplification, particularly of large products. Most studies analyse the gamma T-cell receptor gene which is rearranged in T cells expressing either an alpha-beta or gamma-delta TCR, and this gene can be successfully amplified using a series of four V-gamma family consensus primers and a J-gamma consensus primer, with occasional use of several primers for J-gamma pseudogenes [32]; in contrast, the beta T-cell receptor gene has a very large number of different V-beta family gene segments, which would therefore require a large number of different primers. Thus, because of the large size of the human beta gene, analysis is best performed using cDNA prepared from tumour RNA. RNA is inherently much less stable than DNA and would therefore be difficult in clinical practice. There are a number of studies employing PCR analysis of the gamma TCR gene in cutaneous lymphoproliferative disorders, but interpretation is hampered because a wide variety of electrophoretic methods have been used to analyse the PCR products [15, 33–36]. In addition, most studies have not performed a comprehensive analysis of the gamma TCR gene to fully exclude false-negative results. However, it is clear that the detection sensitivity is at least one order of magnitude greater than Southern blot analysis, with as few as 0.5%–1.0% of tumour cells being detected within a mixed-cell population. The use of single primers rather than multiplex PCR also improves sensitivity, as does the incorporation of radioactivity. Various electrophoretic methods have been employed, including denaturing gradient gel electrophoresis (DGGE) [33], temperature gradient gel electrophoresis (TGGE) [34] and denaturing polyacrylamide gel electrophoresis (PAGE) [15]. We and others have employed the single-strand conformation polymorphism (SSCP) PCR method, which allows comparison of non-denatured and denatured PCR products [35, 36].

Results suggest that T-cell clones can be detected in all stages of mycosis fungoides, with overall detection rates of 53%–75% [33–38]. Our findings suggest a much higher rate of detection, and this may be due to the use of monoplex PCR, employing consensus primers to amplify all possible productive and nonproductive gamma TCR gene rearrangements [35]. Whilst the absence of a clonal rearrangement in a patient with typical early patch-stage mycosis fungoides might be due to a lack of sensitivity, failure to detect a clonal rearrangement in a patient with tumour-stage disease may be due to chromosomal loss involving one or other of the TCR gene loci. It is also important to recognise that analysis of lymphocyte-poor tissues can produce a false-positive result [39], but this is rarely an issue when cutaneous lymphoproliferative disorders are being analysed. Recent studies of DNA extracted from lymph nodes of mycosis fungoides patients has confirmed previous Southern blot findings and shown that T-cell clones can also be detected in lymph nodes graded as LN-1 [40, 41], and that the detection of a T-cell clone in patients with LN-1/LN-2 lymph nodes appears to confer a worse prognosis. Future larger studies should clarify the precise significance of these results. Similarly, peripheral blood T-cell clones can be detected in a much higher percentage of patients with early-stage mycosis fungoides using PCR analysis [34, 35]. Once again, these studies have shown that the T-cell clones are identical to those in skin, but most importantly, the presence of a T-cell clone within peripheral blood in mycosis fungoides is a marker of tumour burden and, critically, an independent prognostic factor [35]. Although studies have shown that peripheral blood T-cell clones can very rarely be detected in healthy elderly individuals over the age of 80 years [42], it is clear that the presence of an identical clonal rearrangement in both peripheral blood and skin of a patient with mycosis fungoides is not likely to be due to a technical artefact or the presence of an unrelated lymphoid clone.

These results indicate that PCR analysis of the gamma T-cell receptor gene can provide independent prognostic information in patients with mycosis fungoides when this approach is used to analyse lymph node and peripheral blood. As such, it will become a critical method of staging patients with mycosis fungoides and will inevitably have therapeutic significance in the future as a reliable marker of tumour burden.

4 Cytogenetic Studies in Cutaneous T-Cell Lymphoma

Conventional karyotypic studies have been restricted mainly to analysis of peripheral blood samples from CTCL patients. Most have involved Sézary syndrome and, to a lesser extent, patients with mycosis fungoides, although not all of the latter group have had documented peripheral blood involvement [43, 44]. These studies have been carried out using conventional mitogen-produced metaphases and there have been few studies of cutaneous tissue, partly because of the difficulty of obtaining good-quality metaphases from solid tumours, the presence of tumour-infiltrating lymphocytes, and an inability to culture tumour cells from patients with CTCL. However, these studies have revealed numerous structural and numerical abnormalities. In some patients nonrandom clonal abnormalities have been detected, but these appear to be patient rather than disease specific, and no consistent chromosomal translocations have been identified. In contrast there is a wealth of literature on other forms of leukaemia and lymphoma, in which disease-specific translocations can provide both diagnostic and prognostic information as well as an insight into the pathogenesis of these malignancies [45]. Nevertheless, recurring abnormalities include chromosomal loss on 1p, rearrangements involving 2p and abnormalities of 10q [43, 44]. In Sézary syndrome abnormal cytogenetic findings are not universal but the presence of an abnormal karyotype is associated with a poor prognosis [46].

Interphase cytogenetics and multicolour FISH analysis (M-FISH) have recently been performed on a small number of CTCL patients [47]. Once again, these studies were done on peripheral blood samples and a variety of numerical and structural abnormalities were identified in patients, including some with early-stage mycosis fungoides and parapsoriasis. Such abnormalities were found more frequently in patient samples than in controls, but it is possible that some of these abnormalities are not disease related. Similarly, numerical and structural abnormalities in late-stage disease may represent chromosomal instability associated with late-stage malignancy. Analysis with M-FISH is a valuable method for characterising chromosomal abnormalities and involves the use of differentially labelled probes for specific chromosomal loci, which allows detailed mapping of chromosomal deletions and translocations. A recent study has also employed a novel method, comparative genomic hybridisation (CGH), which involves differentially labelling tumour DNA and normal lymphocyte DNA, and then competitively hybridising both to normal human metaphases [48]. Complex software analysis of the results enables a global estimation of specific regions of chromosomal gain or loss. This technique has the advantage that tumour DNA can be analysed from skin and lymph node as well as peripheral blood samples. This study identified an abnormal CGH pattern in six of seven Sézary syndrome patients but in none of four patients with mycosis fungoides. In Sézary syndrome, losses were most frequently noted at 10q and 13q [48]. In contrast, gains of chromosome 8q and 17q were also noted. In mycosis fungoides no gains or losses were detected, but four of the Sézary syndrome patients originally had mycosis fungoides with the eventual development of erythrodermic disease. These findings are consistent with previous cytogenetic results and suggest that there are specific chromosomal regions which contain genes involved in the pathogenesis of cutaneous T-cell lymphoma.

5 Candidate Tumour Suppressor Genes

A complementary approach for characterising the underlying molecular abnormalities involved in the pathogenesis of primary cutaneous T-cell lymphomas involves analysis of candidate tumour suppressor genes, which have been implicated in other malignancies. Inactivation of the p53 gene is one of the most common genetic abnormalities currently identified in human malignancy. Studies in non-

Hodgkin's lymphoma have shown evidence of p53 gene inactivation in advanced disease, particularly in aggressive forms such as Burkitt's lymphoma, adult T-cell leukaemia lymphoma associated with HTLV-1, and Richter's transformation in B-CLL [49]. Furthermore, p53 inactivation appears to be associated with treatment resistance in non-Hodgkin's lymphoma [50]. Studies of p53 protein expression in primary cutaneous T-cell lymphoma have shown abnormal expression in late stages of disease [51, 52], but there have been relatively few mutational studies of the p53 gene [53, 54]. Abnormal protein expression can be due to up-regulation of wild-type p53 due to post transcriptional stabilisation or, alternatively, to p53 gene inactivation. Our study of mycosis fungoides identified p53 gene mutations in 40% of patients with tumour-stage disease (stage IIb) but in no patients with early-stage disease [54]. These findings correlated with p53 protein expression. Interestingly, however, the mutation spectrum was consistent with UVB-type mutations. A majority consisted of C-T transitions at dipyrimidine sites, and several CC-TT tandem-base pair transitions were noted. In addition, some of the mutations occurred at hot-spot codons for non-melanoma skin cancer. This type of mutation spectrum is very similar to that found in cutaneous squamous cell carcinoma, which strongly implicates UVB as the cause of these mutations. A number of these patients had received previous phototherapy, but it is impossible at present to establish whether this is an environmental UV effect or related to previous treatment. It is interesting that non-melanoma skin cancer associated with PUVA therapy has also been shown to be associated with UVB-type mutations of p53 [55], suggesting that UVB-type mutations may develop because of concurrent PUVA-induced cutaneous immunosuppression. A recent study of large-cell transformation in mycosis fungoides also identified p53 gene mutations, but the pattern of mutation was not consistent with UVB [56].

A recently proposed controversial hypothesis links the increased incidence of systemic non-Hodgkin's lymphoma with that of increased UV exposure [56]. This is based on a similar increased incidence between non-Hodgkin's lymphoma and non-melanoma skin cancer. It is speculated that this possible link might be due to a systemic immunosuppressive effect of UV rather than an ultraviolet radiation-induced mutation. Epidemiological studies in primary cutaneous lymphoma have not found an association between incidence and latitude in North America [57]. However, our findings suggest that this link would be much more complicated, because the relationship would be between ultraviolet radiation and disease progression. Critically, P53 gene mutations were not detected in early-stage disease, suggesting that this abnormality is associated with disease progression rather than with initiation [54]. While p53 abnormalities in CTCL cannot account solely for a malignant phenotype, there is likely to be considerable clinical relevance. As mentioned previously, there is accumulating evidence that p53 gene inactivation is associated with treatment resistance in non-Hodgkin's lymphoma [50]. Most cancer therapies induce cell death by apoptosis, and p53 is critically involved in control of the cell cycle [58]. Specifically, this provides a mechanism for halting progression of the cell from the G1- into the S-phase of the cycle which allows cells to repair DNA damage prior to proliferation. In addition, p53 can induce cell apoptosis if the extent of DNA damage is too great [58]. A wide variety of different tumour suppressor genes have now been implicated in the pathogenesis of different malignancies. Tumour suppressor genes can be inactivated in three specific ways, namely point mutation/small deletion, promotor gene hypermethylation, or large chromosomal loss/deletion [59]. Different combinations of these mechanisms can inactivate the gene by involvement of both alleles. Allelotyping using highly polymorphic microsatellite markers for different chromosomal regions can identify patterns of loss of heterozygosity, which may define regions of chromosomal deletion. Our recent studies initially focused on 10q because of previous cytogenetic findings and have confirmed that there are two minimal regions of deletion [60]. One certainly inactivates the PTEN tumour suppressor gene, because the use of intragenic microsatellites has confirmed that the PTEN gene is homozygously deleted. However, this does not exclude the possible involvement of other tumour suppressor genes in the same region, and indeed, the second region of minimal deletion harbours a number of candidate genes. Interestingly, loss of heterozygosity on 10q in this study of 51 patients with mycosis fungoides was associated predominantly with disease progression and occurred in 23% of patients overall, suggesting that allelic loss may have prognostic significance [60].

References

1. Bunn P, Lamberg S (1979) Report of the committee on staging and classification of cutaneous T-cell lymphomas. Cancer Treat Rep 63:725–728
2. Bunn P, Huberman M, Whang Peng J, et al. (1980) Prospective staging evaluation of patients with cutaneous T-cell lymphoma. Ann Intern Med 93:223–230
3. Lamberg S, Green S, Byar D, et al. (1984) Clinical staging for cutaneous T-cell lymphoma. Ann Intern Med 100:187–192
4. Willemze R, Kerl H, Sterry W, et al. (1997) EORTC classification for primary cutaneous lymphomas: a proposal from the Cutaneous Lymphoma Study Group of the European Organization for research and treatment of cancer. Blood 90:354–371
5. Sausville E, Eddy J, Makuch R, et al. (1988) Histopathologic staging at initial diagnosis of mycosis fungoides and the Sézary syndrome: definition of three distinctive prognostic groups. Am Intern Med 109:372–382
6. Diamandidou E, Colome M, Fayad L, et al. (1999) Prognostic factor analysis in mycosis fungoides/Sézary syndrome. J Am Acad Dermatol 40:914–924
7. Schechter G, Sausville E, Fischmann A, et al. (1987) Evaluation of circulating malignant cells provides prognostic information in cutaneous T cell lymphoma. Blood 69:841–849
8. Wasik M, Vonderheid E, Bigler R, et al. (1996) Increased serum concentration of the soluble interleukin-2 receptor in cutaneous T-cell lymphoma: clinical and prognostic implications. Arch Dermatol 132:42–47
9. Marti R, Estrach T, Reverter J, et al. (1991) Prognostic clinicopathologic factors in cutaneous T-cell lymphoma. Arch Dermatol 127:1511–1516
10. Alt F, Oltz E, Young F, et al. (1992) VDJ recombination. Immunol Today 13:306–314
11. Asou N, Hattori T, Matsuoka M, et al. (1989) Rearrangements of T-cell antigen receptor and immunoglobulin chain gene in haematologic neoplasms. Blood 74:2707–2712
12. Arnold A, Cossman J, Bakhshi A, et al. (1983) Immunoglobulin gene rearrangements as unique clonal markers in human lymphoid neoplasms. N Engl J Med 309:1593–1599
13. Waldmann T, Davis M, Bongiovanni K et al. (1985) Rearrangements of genes for the antigen receptor on T-cells as markers of lineage and clonality of human lymphoid neoplasms. N Engl J Med 313:776–783
14. Bertness V, Kirsch I, Hollis G, et al. (1985) T-cell receptor gene rearrangements as clinical markers of human T-cell lymphomas. N Engl J Med 313:534–538
15. McCarthy K, Sloane J, Kabarowski J, et al. (1991) The rapid detection of clonal T-cell proliferations in patients with lymphoid disorders. Am J Pathol 138:821–828

16. McCarthy K, Sloane J, Wiedemann L, et al. (1990) Rapid method for distinguishing clonal from polyclonal B cell populations in surgical biopsy specimens. J Clin Pathol 43:429–432
17. Weiss L, Wood G, Trela M, et al. (1986) Clonal T-cell populations in lymphomatoid papulosis. N Engl J Med 315:475–479
18. Whittaker S, Smith N, Russell-Jones R, et al. (1991) Analysis of bb, gg and dd T-cell receptor genes in lymphomatoid papulosis: cellular basis of two distinct histologic subsets. J Invest Dermatol 96:786–791
19. Headington J, Roth M, Ginsberg D, et al. (1987) T-cell receptor gene rearrangement in regressing atypical histiocytosis. Arch Dermatol 123:1183–1187
20. Wood G, Weiss L, Hu C, et al. (1988) T-cell antigen deficiencies and clonal rearrangements of T-cell receptor genes in pagetoid reticulosis (Woringer-Kolopp disease). N Engl J Med 318:164–167
21. LeBoit P, Becksteid J, Bond B, et al. (1987) Granulomatous slack skin: clonal rearrangement of the T-cell receptor β gene is evidence for the lymphoproliferative nature of a cutaneous elastolytic disorder. J Invest Dermatol 89:183–186
22. LeBoit P, Abel A, Cleary M, et al. (1988) Clonal circulating T-cells in erythrodermic follicular mucinosis. Blood 71:1329–33
23. Weiss L, Hu E, Wood G et al. (1985b) Clonal rearrangements of T-cell receptor genes in mycosis fungoides and dermatopathic lymphadenopathy. N Engl J Med 313:539–544
24. Whittaker S, Smith N, Russell-Jones R, et al. (1991) Analysis of β, γ and δ T-cell receptor genes in mycosis fungoides and Sézary syndrome. Cancer 68:1572–1582
25. Lynch J, Linoilla I, Sausville E, et al. (1992) Prognostic implications of evaluation for lymph node involvement by T-cell antigen receptor gene rearrangement in mycosis fungoides. Blood 79:3293–3299
26. Bakels V, Van Oostveen J, Geerts S, et al. (1993) Diagnostic and prognostic significance of clonal T-cell receptor beta gene rearrangements in lymph nodes of patients with mycosis fungoides. J Pathol 170:249–255
27. Weiss L, Wood G, Hu C, et al. (1989) Detection of clonal T-cell receptor gene rearrangements in the peripheral blood of patients with mycosis fungoides/Sézary syndrome. J Invest Dermatol 92:601–604
28. Bagot M, Wechsler J, Lescs M, et al. (1992) Intra-epidermal localisation of the clone in cutaneous T-cell lymphoma. J Am Acad Dermatol 27:589–593
29. Bahler D, Berry G, Oksenberg J, et al. (1992) Diversity of T-cell antigen receptor variable genes used by mycosis fungoides cells. Am J Pathol 140:1–8
30. Bogen S, Pelley D, Charif M, et al. (1996) Immunophenotypic identification of Sézary cells in peripheral blood. Am J Clin Pathol 106:739–748
31. Bernengo M, Quaglino P, Novelli M, et al. (1998) Prognostic factors in Sézary syndrome: a multivariate analysis of clinical, haematological and immunological features. Ann Oncol 9:857–863
32. Theodorou I, Raphaël M, Bigorgne C, et al. (1994) Recombination pattern of the TCR γ locus in human peripheral T-cell lymphomas. J Pathol 174:233–242
33. Wood G, Tung R, Haeffner A, et al. (1994) Detection of clonal T-cell receptor γ gene rearrangements in early mycosis fungoides/Sézary syndrome by polymerase chain reaction and denaturing gradient gel electrophoresis (PCR/DGGE). J Invest Dermatol 103: 34–41
34. Muche J, Lukowsky A, Asadullah K, et al. (1997) Demonstration of frequent occurrence of clonal T cells in the peripheral blood of patients with primary cutaneous T-cell lymphoma. Blood 90:1636–1642
35. Fraser-Andrews E, Woolford A, Russell-Jones R, et al. (2000) Detection of a peripheral blood T-cell clone is an independent prognostic marker in mycosis fungoides. J Invest Dermatol 114:117–121
36. Bottaro M, Berti E, Biondi A, et al. (1994) Heteroduplex analysis of T-cell receptor γ gene rearrangements for diagnosis and monitoring of cutaneous T-cell lymphomas. Blood 83:3271–3278
37. Davis T, Yockey C, Balk S (1993) Detection of clonal immunoglobulin gene rearrangements by polymerase chain reaction amplification and single strand conformational polymorphism analysis. Am J Pathol 142:1841–1847

38. Boehncke W, Krettek S, Parwaresch M, et al. (1992) Demonstration of clonal disease in early mycosis fungoides. Am J Dermatopathol 14:95–9
39. Ling F, Clark C, Lillicrap D (1992) Positive immunoglobulin gene rearrangement study by the polymerase chain reaction in a colonic adenocarcinoma. Am J Pathol 98:116–119
40. Kern D, Kidd P, Moe R, et al. (1998) Analysis of T-cell receptor gene rearrangement in lymph nodes of patients with mycosis fungoides. Arch Dermatol 134:158–164
41. Lynch J jr, Linoilla I, Sausville E, et al. (1992) Prognostic implications of evaluation of lymph node involvement by T-cell antigen receptor gene rearrangement in mycosis fungoides. Blood 79:3293–3299
42. Posnett D, Sinha R, Kabak S, et al. (1994) Clonal populations of T-cells in normal elderly humans: the T-cell equivalent to "Benign monoclonal gammapathy". J Exp Med 179:609–618
43. Limon J, Nedosztko B, Brozek I, et al. (1995) Chromosome aberrations, spontaneous SCE and growth kinetics in PHA-stimulated lymphocytes in 5 cases of Sézary syndrome. Cancer Genet Cytogenet 83:75
44. Thangavelu M, Finn W, Yelavarthi K, et al. (1997) Recurring structural chromosomal abnormalities in peripheral blood lymphocytes of patients with mycosis fungoides/Sézary syndrome. Blood 89:3371
45. Rabbitts T (1991) Translocations, master genes, and differences between the origins of acute and chronic leukaemias. Cell 67:641–644
46. Berger R, Bernheim A (1987) Cytogenetic studies of Sézary cells. Cancer Genet Cytogenet 27:79–87
47. Karenko L, Hyytinen E, Sarna S, et al. (1997) Chromosomal abnormalities in cutaneous T-cell lymphoma and in its premalignant conditions as detected by G-banding and interphase cytogenetic methods. J Invest Dermatol 108–122
48. Karenko L, Kahkonen M, Hyytinen E, et al. (1999) Notable losses at specific regions of chromosome 10q and 13q in the Sézary syndrome detected by comparative genomic hybridisation. J Invest Dermatol 112–392
49. Galdano G, Ballerini P, Gong J, et al. (1991) p53 Mutations in human lymphoid malignancies: association with Burkitt lymphoma and chronic lymphocytic leukaemia. Proc Natl Acad Sci USA 88:5413–5417
50. Wilson W, Teruya-Feldstein J, Fest T, et al. (1997) Relationship of p53, bcl-2, and tumour proliferation to clinical drug resistance in non-Hodgkin's lymphomas. Blood 89:601–609
51. Lauritzen A, Vejlsgaard G, Hou-Jensen K, et al. (1995) p53 protein expression in cutaneous T-cell lymphomas. Br J Dermatol 133:32–36
52. McGregor J, Dublin E, Levison D, et al. (1995) p53 immunoreactivity is uncommon in primary cutaneous lymphoma. Br J Dermatol 132:353
53. Marks D, Vonderheid E, Kurz B, et al. (1996) Analysis of p53 and mdm-2 expression in 18 patients with Sézary syndrome. Br J Haematol 92:890–899
54. McGregor J, Crook T, Fraser-Andrews E, et al. (1999) Spectrum of p53 gene mutations suggests a possible role for ultraviolet radiation in the pathogenesis of advanced cutaneous lymphomas. J Invest Dermatol 112:317–321
55. Nataraj A, Wolf P, Cerroni L, et al. (1997) p53 mutation in squamous cell carcinomas from psoriasis patients treated with psoralen + UVA (PUVA). J Invest Dermatol 109:238–243
56. Cartwright R, McNally R, Staines A (1994) The increasing incidence of non-Hodgkin's lymphoma (NHL): the possible role of sunlight. Leuk Lymphoma 14:387–394
57. Newton R (1997) Solar ultraviolet radiation is not a major cause of primary cutaneous non-Hodgkin's lymphomas. Br Med J 314:1483–1484
58. Lane D (1992) Cancer. P53, guardian of the genome. Nature 358:15–16
59. Jones P, Laird P (1999) Cancer epigenetics comes of age. Nat Genet 21:163–167
60. Scarisbrick J, Woolford A, Russell-Jones R, et al. (2000) Loss of heterozygosity on 10q and microsatellite instability in advanced stages of primary cutaneous T-cell lymphoma and possible association with homozygous deletion of PTEN. Blood 95:2937–2942

Skin Lesions of Fibrocytic and Fibrohistiocytic Differentiation: A New Concept and Classification

B. G. Zelger, B. Zelger

1 Introduction

The WHO classification of soft-tissue tumours derives from an article in a fascicle of the AFIP atlas in 1953 by Arthur Purdy Stout [1], the leading specialist on soft-tissue neoplasia at that time, and was later modified several times. Its current version [2] differentiates entities according to their histopathological derivation into 15 different groups, among them fibrous and fibrohistiocytic tumours, and further subdivides both of these according to their biological behaviour into benign, intermediate, and malignant lesions (Table 1). However, there are great difficulties with this classification, for several reasons.

Firstly, pathology in general and dermatopathology in particular, which both evaluate sections fixed by formalin and embedded in paraffin, cannot reliably re-

Current Topics in Pathology
Volume 94; R. Cerio (Ed.)

Table 1. WHO classification of fibrous and fibrohistiocytic tumours [2]

1	Fibrous tissue tumours
1.1	Benign
1.1.1	Fibroma
1.1.2	Keloid
1.1.3	Nodular fasciitis
1.1.4	Proliferative fasciitis, proliferative myositis
1.1.5	Elastofibroma
1.1.6	Fibrous hamartoma of infancy
1.1.7	Myofibromatosis, solitary and multicentric
1.1.8	Fibromatosis colli
1.1.9	Calcifying aponeurotic fibroma
1.1.10	Hyaline fibromatosis
1.2	Fibromatosis
1.2.1	Superficial fibromatosis
1.2.1.1	Palmar and plantar fibromatosis
1.2.1.2	Infantile digital fibromatosis (digital fibroma)
1.2.2	Deep fibromatosis
1.2.2.1	Abdominal fibromatosis (desmoid tumour)
1.2.2.2	Extra-abdominal fibromatosis (desmoid tumour)
1.2.2.3	Intra-abdominal and mesenteric fibromatosis
1.2.2.4	Infantile fibromatosis
1.3	Malignant
1.3.1	Fibrosarcoma
1.3.1.1	Adult fibrosarcoma
1.3.1.2	Congenital or infantile fibrosarcoma
2	Fibrohistiocytic tumours
2.1	Benign
2.1.1	Fibrous histiocytoma
2.1.1.1	Cutaneous histiocytoma (dermatofibroma)
2.1.1.2	Deep histiocytoma
2.1.2	Juvenile xanthogranuloma
2.1.3	Reticulohistiocytoma
2.1.4	Xanthoma
2.2	Intermediate
2.2.1	Atypical fibroxanthoma
2.2.2	Dermatofibrosarcoma protuberans, pigmented dermatofibrosarcoma protuberans (Bednar tumour)
2.2.3	Giant cell fibroblastoma
2.2.4	Plexiform fibrohistiocytic tumour
2.2.5	Angiomatoid fibrous histiocytoma
2.3	Malignant
2.3.1	Malignant fibrous histiocytoma
2.3.1.1	Storiform pleomorphic
2.3.1.2	Myxoid
2.3.1.3	Giant cell
2.3.1.4	Xanthomatous (inflammatory)

cognise histogenesis, but only evaluate what differentiation a lesion shows, and such differentiation may vary. For example, early lesions of dermatofibroma [3] may be rich in "histiocytes" and have accordingly been named histiocytoma (cutis) or fibrous histiocytoma. In contrast, long-standing lesions of dermatofibroma consist mostly of fibrocytes and collagen and have in the past been termed fibroma durum, subepidermal nodular fibrosis or sclerosis, and more currently sclerotic or sclerosing fibroma. Basically, it is the same process, a fibrosing dermatitis [3], visualised at different moments of its life history, and what is meant by histiocytic differentiation is the presence of macrophages with phagocytic properties within these lesions. Moreover, the concept of histiocytes (from the Greek "τὸ ἵστιον", for "tissue", i.e. cells in the tissue, in contrast to epithelium) is also flawed [4]: there are many more cells than just macrophages in the tissue, such as fibrocytes, mast cells, endothelial cells, nerve cells, and smooth muscle cells.

Secondly, when the WHO classification [2] mentions tumours it really means neoplasms, either benign or malignant. However, tumour is a descriptive term which characterises circumscribed lesions with a diameter larger than 2 cm (skin lesions smaller than 1 cm are papules, those between 1 and 2 cm nodules). According to this definition, most dermatofibromas, nearly all xanthogranulomas, many atypical fibroxanthomas and some "early" sarcomas (smaller than 2 cm in maximum diameter) would fall outside the category of tumours. Moreover, the term tumour gives no information about the nature of its underlying process. Tumours may be neoplastic, either benign as in fibroma of tendon sheath or malignant as in dermatofibrosarcoma protuberans, inflammatory such as in keloids, hyperplastic as in prurigo, or hamartomatous such as in connective tissue nevi, to mention but a few examples. As we see it, only a minority of entities listed in the WHO classification are real neoplasms, either benign or malignant.

Thirdly, the subdivision of entities into benign, intermediate, and malignant is an attempt to overcome a clinicopathological problem inherent in the making of a histopathological diagnosis: We can never predict the clinical outcome, i.e. the biological behaviour, of a malignant neoplasm. On the one hand, atypical fibroxanthoma – which histopathologically is a clearly malignant lesion with an asymmetrical silhouette, sheets of storiform-pleomorphic tumour cells and numerous, frequently atypical mitoses – will in the vast majority of cases be cured by simple excision; such lesions have in the past been termed "pseudomalignancies" [4]. Nevertheless, there are rare cases of atypical fibroxanthoma which have metastasised and killed the patient [5]. On the other hand, deep fibromatoses (desmoid tumours), which histopathologically have a seemingly bland cytologic appearance, may, when incompletely excised, recur and recur [6] and eventually "progress" to fibrosarcoma [7]. Such lesions fall into a group termed "pseudobenignancies" [4]. The creation of an additional category of intermediate neoplasms between clearly benign and clearly malignant lesions is intended to justify these clinicopathological phenomena. It is simply another frustrating attempt to predict biological behaviour on the basis of histopathological criteria. Moreover, vague terminology such as "pseudomalignancies" or "pseudobenignancies" is not consistently used and thus carries a risk of causing damage to the patient. Dermatofibroma with monster cells and pseudosarcomatous dermatofibroma are examples of "pseudomalignancies" which will never cause any problem to the patient affected by them; they are just a histopathological curiosity and do not require further or even wide excisions.

Finally, the present WHO classification of soft-tissue tumours in general and fibrous/fibrohistiocytic tumours in particular lumps together heterogeneous entities. For example, the intermediate group of fibrous tumours, the so-called fibromatoses [2], consists of superficial and deep variants. Whereas representatives of the superficial group such as Dupuytren's contracture, Ledderhose's disease and Peyronie's disease are fibrosing inflammatory disorders which, apart from local functional impairment, never cause any further serious problems, deep fibromatoses (desmoid tumours) are low-grade malignancies prone to frequent recurrences and occasional metastases [7]. While infantile fibromatosis is listed together with these entities as a fibromatosis, myofibromatosis (solitary and multicentric), fibromatosis colli, and hyaline fibromatosis are incorporated in the benign group of fibrous tissue tumours. Lumping together of such heterogeneous entities on the one hand and splitting them into different groups of classification systems on the other cannot promote our understanding of these disorders. Moreover, multicentric myofibromatosis (as well as solitary myofibroma) reveals pericytic differentiation with a haemangiopericytoma-like pattern in early stages, and leiomyoma-like features in later stages. These features are not seen in lesions of fibroblastic differentiation.

Classical pathology subdivides diseases into seven groups [8]: hamartomas, malformations, hyperplasias, inflammatory disorders, benign and malignant neoplasms, cysts and deposits. *Hamartoma* (from the Greek "ἁμαρτάνομαι" for "to err") defines lesions, frequently congenital, sometimes developing during later life (tardive), which consist of an abnormal composition of tissue components physiologically inherent to a certain region such as naevus sebaceous or congenital melanocytic naevi. In contrast to neoplasms, their growth is not independent of, but parallels the growth of the host patient or surrounding structures. *Malformations* are abnormal structures deriving from incorrect development of the "embryonal anlage", such as craniofacial dysplasias, meningoceles ("glioma nasi") or arteriovenous shunts, and are frequently mixed up synonymously with hamartomas. *Hyperplasia* is an increase in number of cells (in contrast to hypertrophy, where the size of the single cell is increased, e.g. in muscular hypertrophy) which waxes and wanes with the presence of such stimuli as rubbing in prurigo nodules, human papilloma virus in warts, or iodine in thyroid adenomas. *Inflammatory diseases* consist of an infiltrate of inflammatory cells only. In contrast, *neoplastic diseases* are composed, at least in part, of cells other than inflammatory cells, i.e. neoplastic cells. Benign and malignant neoplasms differ by their limited or unlimited autonomous growth, capable of killing the patient by local invasion or distant metastases in the latter case. The term neoplasm is deliberately preferred to the less-specific term tumour (see above), which is frequently also applied to non-neoplastic disorders such as cysts (e.g. pilomatricoma), deposits (e.g. tophus) or inflammatory disorders (e.g. dermatofibroma). Moreover, neoplasms may present not only as tumours, but also as macules, papules or plaques such as the macular or flat lesions of melanoma ("lentigo maligna" or "superficial spreading melanoma"). *Cysts* are sac-like spaces filled with liquid or nonliquid substances produced by the epithelial lining . Finally, *deposits* stem from metabolic disorders that lead to the deposition of various substances within the tissue. This review adopts the above classification for fibrocytic and fibrohistiocytic lesions in skin (see Table 2).

Table 2. Lesions of fibrocytic and fibrohistiocytic differentiation: a new concept and classification

1	Inflammatory disorders
1.1	Scars
1.2	Keloids
1.3	Dermatofibroma
1.4	Nodular fasciitis
1.5	Superficial fibromatoses
1.6	Xanthogranuloma
2	Hyperplasias
2.1	Prurigo nodularis
2.2	Knuckle pads
3	Hamartomas
3.1	Fibroma molle
3.2	Fibrous papules
2.3	Connective-tissue naevi
2.4	Elastofibroma
4	Benign neoplasms
4.1	Fibroma of tendon sheath
4.2	Pleomorphic fibroma
4.3	Giant cell tumour of tendon sheath
5	Malignant neoplasms
5.1	Dermatofibrosarcoma protuberans
5.2	Myxofibrosarcoma (myxoid malignant fibrous histiocytoma)
5.3	Fibrosarcoma
5.4	Deep fibromatoses (desmoid fibromatoses, desmoids)
5.5	Solitary fibrous tumour

2 Inflammatory Disorders

Fibrosing dermatitis [3] is the reaction pattern most commonly associated with inflammatory lesions of fibrocytic and fibrohistiocytic differentiation such as (hypertrophic) scars, keloids, most variants of dermatofibroma and superficial fibromatoses. Yet the algorithmic approach of histopathological diagnosis of inflammatory skin diseases with fibrocytic and fibrohistiocytic differentiation [3] may follow other reaction patterns such as a nodular to diffuse dermatitis in xanthogranulomas, subepidermal vesicular dermatitis in early scar formation, perifolliculitis in some forms of dermatofibromas or panniculitis in nodular fasciitis. Clinicopathologically, six groups of inflammatory fibrocytic and fibrohistiocytic disorders can be distinguished.

2.1 Scars

Clinically, scars [3] can occur at any age or location and in either sex. Usually lesions are localised, but sometimes they are widespread, e.g. following acne. Scars are mostly linear as in surgical wounds, but they may also be round as a consequence of an ulcer induced factitiously, bizarre as in white atrophy, diffuse following dermabrasion, or punctate as the "ice-pick" scars of acne vulgaris. Individual lesions may present as papules, plaques, nodules, or atrophic macules and patches. Clinical variations include hypertrophic scars such as burn scars and those following surgical incisions, or atrophic scars such as those of macular atrophy in acne vulgaris. Differential diagnosis includes dermatofibroma, an oval to round, hyperpigmented lesion which dimples when squeezed between the fingers; keloids extend beyond the boundary of the original wound and do not shrink considerably over a period of years.

Histologically (Fig. 1), early lesions show granulation tissue; fully developed lesions show thin bundles of collagen and plump fibrocytes oriented parallel to the skin surface, dilated venules situated mostly perpendicular to the skin surface, variable mucin and an absence of elastic fibres. Late lesions are similar to those in fully developed lesions, but with thicker collagen bundles and less prominent fibrocytes and blood vessels. Differential diagnosis includes keloids, which exhibit markedly thickened, brightly eosinophilic bundles of collagen arranged haphazardly, and dermatofibroma, which shows randomly arranged histiocytes, fibrocytes and coarse bundles of collagen with prominent peripheral collagen, as well as variable epidermal, melanocytic and folliculosebaceous hyperplasia above the lesions.

a 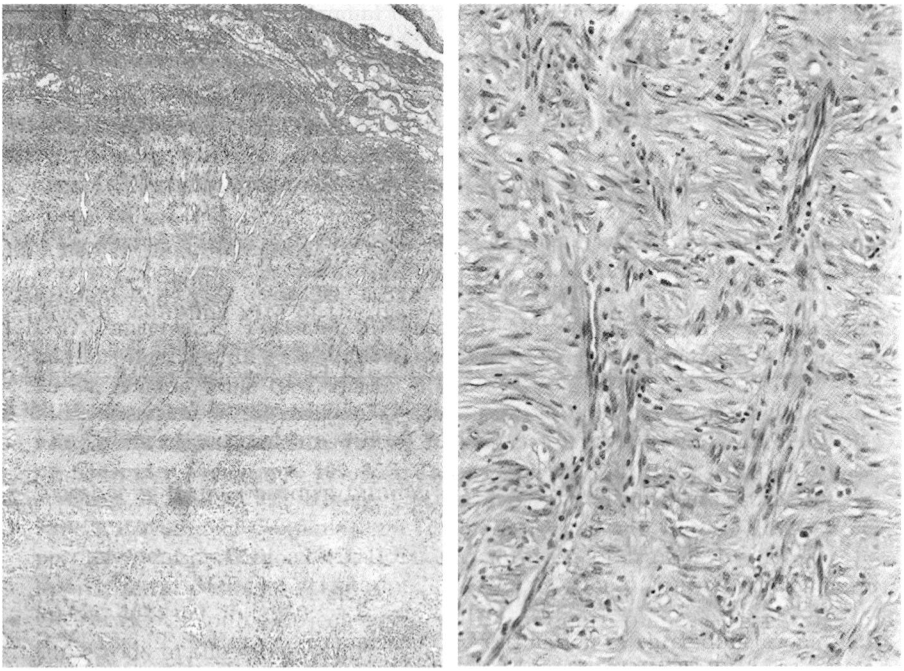 b

Fig. 1a, b. Scar: **a** Granulation tissue with vessels perpendicular to ulcerated surface and (**b**) horizontally aligned fibroblasts beside delicate collagen bundles

2.2 Keloids

Clinically, keloids [3] preferentially affect young adults of either sex, and they are more often seen in darkly pigmented individuals. The sternal region, ear lobes, shoulders, and upper part of the trunk are the preferred sites of characteristic lesions with claw-like extensions at the periphery. Individual lesions may present as papules, plaques, nodules and tumours. Differential diagnosis includes hypertrophic scars which do not extend beyond the boundary of the original wound and tend to shrink considerably over a period of years.

Histologically (Fig. 2), early lesions show granulation tissue and fibroplasia similar to a hypertrophic scar, yet randomly placed; fully developed lesions have numerous thick, brightly eosinophilic bundles of collagen in a random fashion, plump fibrocytes oriented parallel to the course of collagen bundles, and prominent mucin in spaces between collagen bundles; late lesions are similar to fully developed lesions, but have thicker collagen bundles, fewer plump fibrocytes, and less mucin. Differential diagnosis includes hypertrophic scars without markedly thickened bundles of collagen; dermatofibromas with granulomatous features such as siderophages and lipophages and variable epidermal, melanocytic and folliculosebaceous hyperplasia above the lesions.

a
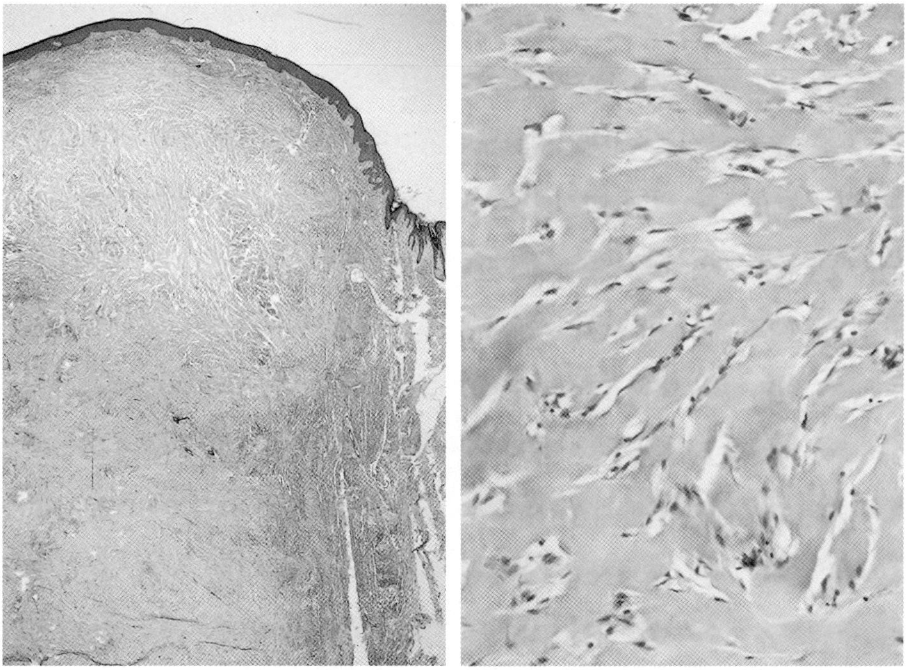
b

Fig. 2a, b. Keloid: **a** Exoendophytic ill-defined nodule (**b**) with sclerotic collagen bundles aligned by bland fibroblasts

2.3 Dermatofibroma

Clinically, dermatofibroma [3] may present at any age and location and in either sex, but it preferentially affects young females, usually on the extremities, in particular the legs and thighs. Usually, a dermatofibroma is a single, round, oval to "targetoid" papule; occasionally there may be a few, sometimes grouped ("agminated") papules, e.g. multinucleate cell angiohistiocytoma, or lesions may form plaques, nodules or tumours, e.g. giant dermatofibromas. Early lesions are reddish, older are brown to skin-coloured. The "dimpling" sign when lesions are squeezed between the fingers is characteristic. Differential diagnosis includes keloids, which are on the chest or ear lobes, tend to be larger, and have claw-like extensions and a more shiny surface; Spitz naevi, which are more red, more common in children on the face and hands, and not firm unless they are mostly intradermal and desmoplastic; and dermatofibrosarcoma protuberans, an irregular lesion that varies in size, shape, colour, surface and consistency and will continue to grow slowly, but consistently, over years to decades.

Histologically (Fig. 3), early lesions show a dense diffuse infiltrate of mostly histiocytes (often both lipophages and siderophages) with numerous extravasated erythrocytes in the reticular dermis and, sometimes, the upper part of the subcutis. Histiocytes at the periphery splay between thickened bundles of col-

a

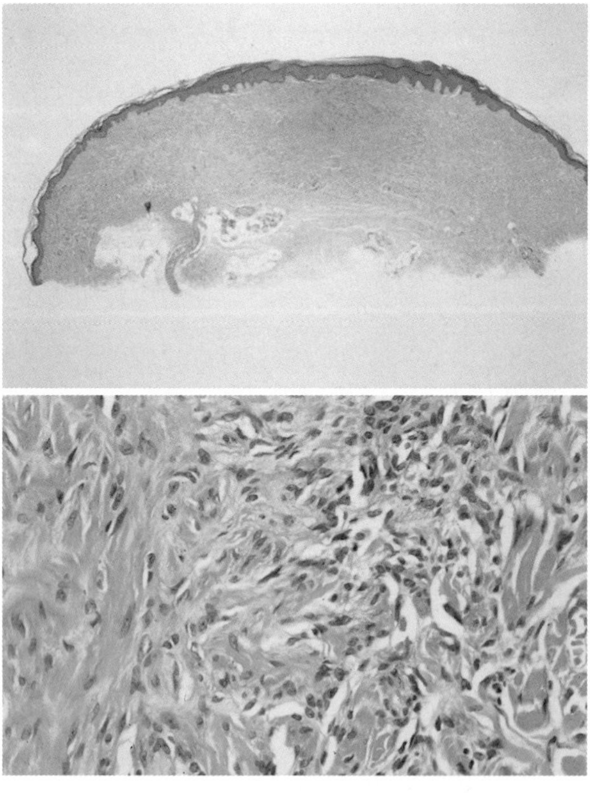

b

Fig. 3 a, b. Dermatofibroma: **a** Characteristic silhouette of spindle cell lesion (**b**) with haphazard, coarse collagen bundles ("storiform pattern")

lagen, vascularity is prominent, and epidermal hyperplasia and hyperpigmentation may be present. Fully developed lesions reveal a dense diffuse infiltrate of histiocytes, some of which may be siderophages and/or lipophages, others multinucleate, e.g. Touton giant cells, or in rare cases with striking pleomorphism of the nuclei, as well as numerous fibrocytes; histiocytes and fibrocytes splay between markedly thickened collagen bundles at the periphery of the lesion and epidermal, melanocytic and folliculosebaceous hyperplasia is found above the lesions. A variable number of lymphocytes are spread diffusely throughout the lesion, with frequent prominence at the periphery. At times, foam cells may be prominent in deeper parts of the lesions adjacent to subcutaneous fat. Late lesions show prominence of fibrocytes and coarse bundles of collagen in a haphazard fashion, sometimes arranged in short fascicles that interweave ("storiform"). At the periphery fibrocytes are splayed between thickened collagen bundles; the centre may sometimes be sclerotic, and epidermal, melanocytic and folliculosebaceous hyperplasia are sparse or absent as are lymphocytes within and around the lesions.

The clinicopathological appearance varies according to the age, size, and site of the lesion, the location within the dermis, the preponderance of particular histological components, and the arrangement of individual or multiple lesions. Each of these lesions may cause characteristic diagnostic difficulties, and for this reason a wide variety of dermatofibromas has been propagated [9]. Early lesions may be red because of proliferation of blood vessels, e.g. known as *sclerosing haemangiomas*, or violaceous because of the extravasation of erythrocytes. When blood is extravasated in large quantities, pre-existing lesions increase suddenly, may hurt, become blue or even black, and may be confused clinically with angiomas or even melanomas, or histologically with nodular stages of Kaposi's sarcoma, e.g. in *aneurysmal* or *angiomatoid fibrous histiocytoma*. Later, the papule becomes yellow or brown, depending on the proportion of lipophages and siderophages in the dense dermal infiltrate, known as *fibrous xanthoma*, or *elusive/haemosiderrhotic dermatofibroma*. Later still, the papule becomes hard; it is then known as *dermatofibroma, fibrous histiocytoma, subepidermal nodular fibrosis, subepidermal nodular sclerosis,* or *fibroma durum*. In time, shrinkage of fibroplasia may flatten the lesion, which becomes thinner than the surrounding dermis, e.g. in *atrophic dermatofibromas*, which frequently occur in the shoulder girdle of young adult women and are clinically misdiagnosed as basal cell carcinoma. Large lesions ("giant dermatofibroma") may cause exoendophytic nodules or tumours, e.g. in *deep penetrating dermatofibroma*, or large flat plaques up to more than 20 cm in diameter, e.g. in *dermatomyofibroma* or *plaque-like dermal fibromatosis* [10], all of which may be confused with dermatofibrosarcoma protuberans, in particular its plaque-like variant in the latter instance. In contrast, small dermatofibromas restricted to the papillary dermis are known as *epithelioid cell histiocytomas* (Fig. 4). Clinically, these exophytic papules frequently reveal a pigmented rim which is due to prominent epidermal hyperplasia and hyperpigmentation ("collarette)"; such lesions have sheet-like infiltrates of epithelioid histiocytes with scalloped cell borders and may be confused with Spitz naevi. Similar histiocytes in a whorled array are found in *cellular neurothekeomas* (Fig. 5), according to our experience [11], a plexiform variant of epithelioid cell histiocytoma in the reticular dermis; cellular neurothekeomas frequently show transition to areas with

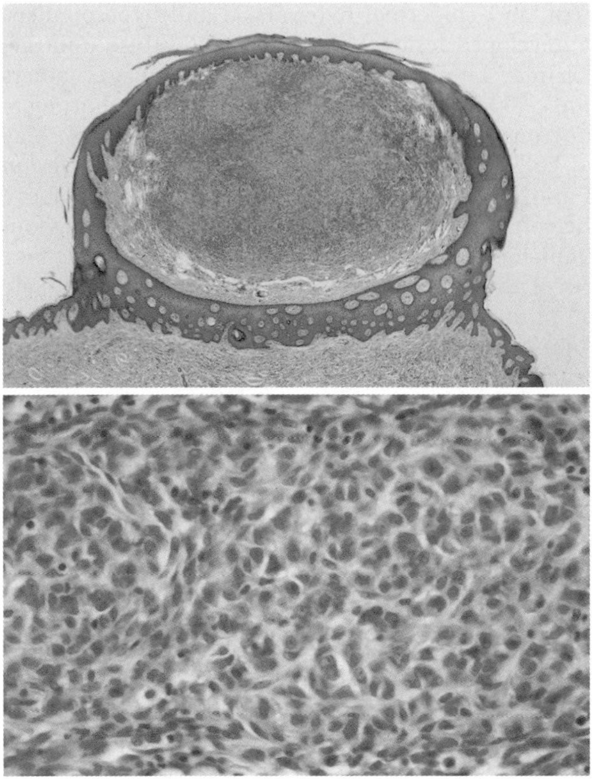

a

b

Fig. 4a, b. Epithelioid cell histiocytoma: **a** Exophytic papule with epidermal collarette and (**b**) sheets of epithelioid histiocytes

features more commonly associated with dermatofibromas and are completely unrelated to myxoid neurothekeomas (nerve sheath myxomas), a myxoid variant of plexiform schwannoma. Other unusual features which are more usually associated with dermatofibromas include monster cells, osteoclast-like giant cells with calcification and/or ossification on the one hand and dense cellularity on the other. The former are known as *dermatofibromas with monster cells* and *ossifying dermatofibroma* and may be misinterpreted as being atypical fibroxanthomas or extraskeletal osteosarcoma, respectively. The latter are described as *pseudosarcomatous/atypical fibrous histiocytomas* and *cellular benign fibrous histiocytoma;* they may, when incompletely excised, occasionally recur and then cause diagnostic difficulties, in particular, in differentiation from leiomyosarcoma and sarcomatous dermatofibrosarcoma protuberans. Further peculiarities arise from strange cytologic features such as granular or clear cell changes, which can cause them to be misinterpreted as classic granular cell schwannoma or metastases of renal cell carcinoma, respectively. Or dermatofibromas may show myofibroblastic differentiation with extremely slender cytoplasmic cell extensions and a strong reactivity for smooth muscle-specific actin. In these cases one speaks of *granular cell, clear cell*, and *myofibroblastic dermatofibromas*, respectively. Stromal peculiarities include prominent sclerosis in *sclerotic fibroma/storiform collagenoma*, which is purported to be an episodic expression of Cowden's disease; excessive mucin

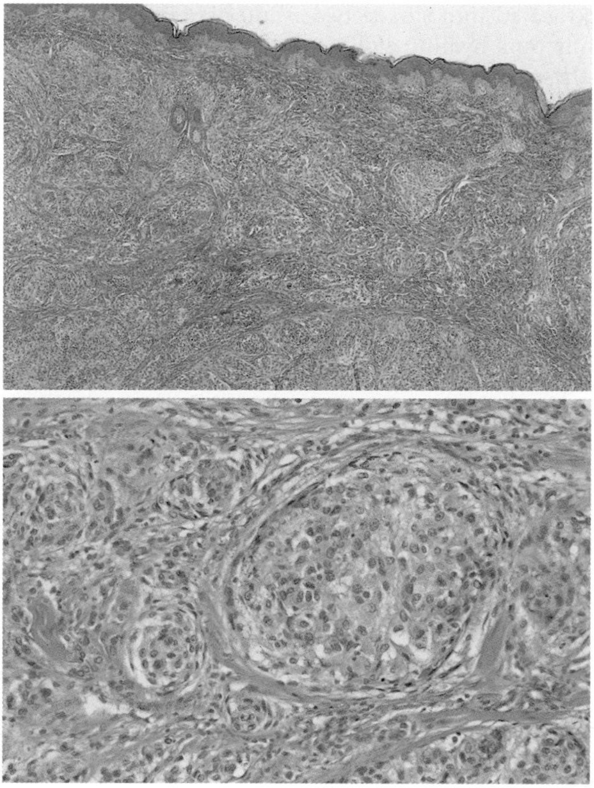

a

b

Fig. 5 a, b. Cellular neurothekeoma: **a** Ill-defined plexiform lesion (**b**) with whorled nests of epithelioid histiocytes beside coarse collagen bundles

deposits in *myxoid dermatofibromas*, lesions frequently misinterpreted as myxomas or mucous cysts [12]; cholesterotic deposits in *cholesterotic fibrous histiocytoma* may mimic gout or prominent palisading in *palisading fibrous histiocytoma* schwannomas. In *multinucleate cell angiohistiocytoma* [10] several to numerous papules of dermatofibroma in a grouped ("agminated") arrangement, mostly on the trunk and proximal extremities, are frequently mistaken for Kaposi's sarcoma or sarcoidosis. Histology reveals prominent ectatic vessels with bizarre giant cells in a fibrosclerotic stroma with moderate epidermal and melanocytic hyperplasia above the lesions. Apart from all these individual peculiarities some lesions may show a combination of several unusual histopathological features; recognition of such *combined dermatofibromas* [13] allows the histopathologist to apply a confident benign label to unusual lesions which might otherwise elude diagnosis, or tempt him or her to describe "new" entities, and to avoid a misdiagnosis of malignancy.

Differential diagnosis includes, firstly, dermatofibrosarcoma protuberans, a poorly circumscribed lesion that is usually much broader and deeper with irregular dissection of the subcutis and shows cells with wavy nuclei in association with delicate fibrillary bundles of collagen frequently arranged in a storiform pattern. In contrast to dermatofibroma, dermatofibrosarcoma protuberans is positive for CD34. Secondly, Kaposi's sarcoma in the nodular and tumour stage is characterised by erythrocytes extravasated into slits between interweaving fascicles of spindle-shaped cells; often, tiny pink hyaline globules that represent degenerated erythrocytes are found in these spindle-shaped endothelial cells. Lesions are positive for *Ulex europaeus* agglutinin, as well as for vascular markers such as factor VIII, CD31 and CD34.

2.4 Nodular Fasciitis

Nodular fasciitis [4] is in the subcutis what dermatofibroma represents in the papillary and/or reticular dermis, i. e. a fibrosing panniculitis. Clinically, nodular fasciitis preferentially affects young adults of either sex; it is localised to the extremities, mostly the forearms, and the upper trunk in adults, but in the head and neck in children. Individual lesions present as nodules, and as tumours which frequently evolve rapidly within one to several weeks and resolve slowly within months. Differential diagnosis includes metastases to the skin, which usually occur on the scalp of older people, are better circumscribed and harder than nodular fasciitis.

Histologically (Fig. 6), at scanning magnification, lesions are moderately well circumscribed, with either a round to oval or an irregular stellate appearance. Early

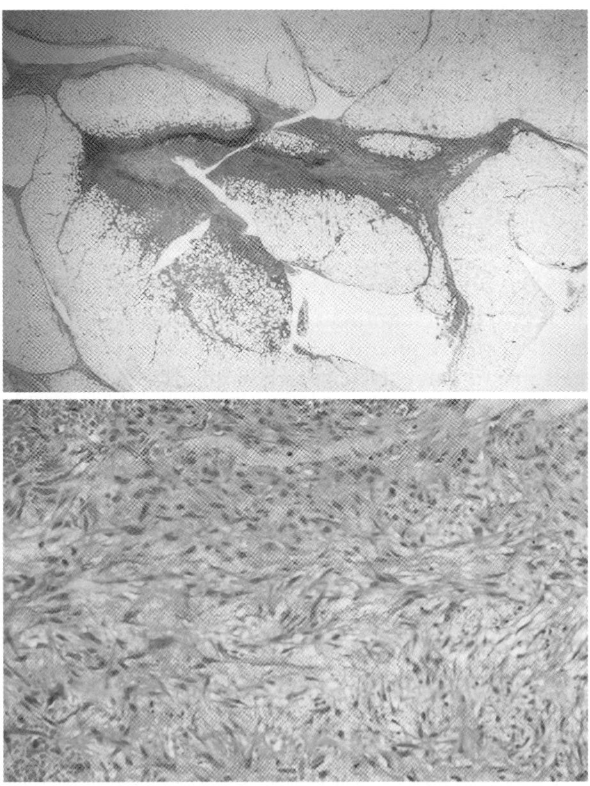

a

b

Fig. 6 a, b. Nodular fasciitis: **a** Ill-defined stellate subcutaneous lesion (**b**) with tissue-culture-like appearance of fibroblasts

lesions show granulation tissue and fibroplasia similar to a hypertrophic scar, but in haphazard array in the subcutis, within and above or below the fascia in the striated muscles; fully developed lesions show fibroplasia accompanying granulation tissue, plump fibrocytes with large oval nuclei and sometimes elongated extensions of cytoplasm, oriented parallel to the course of collagen bundles, some multinucleate giant cells, and prominent mucin in spaces between collagen bundles. The cytologic appearance of fibrocytes together with prominent mucin is characteristic of the so-called feathery or tissue culture-like appearance of these lesions; late lesions are similar to fully developed lesions, but with fibroplasia and sclerosis increasing as granulation tissue, fibrocytes, and mucin decrease and the lesion as a whole shrinks. Differential diagnosis includes first fibrosarcoma which exhibits herringbone-like fascicles with cellular atypia, but usually less mucin and inflammatory cells. In addition, necrotising fasciitis can be ruled out by the absence of thrombosis of subcutaneous vessels and suppuration.

According to the variable location [6], lesions have been called *parosteal, cranial,* or *intravascular fasciitis,* or *proliferative myositis*; similarly, according to the variable histopathological presentation [6], synonyms such as pseudosarcomatous, proliferative, infiltrative, or ossifying fasciitis; pseudosarcomatous fibromatosis; panniculitis, fasciitis and myositis ossificans have been used in the literature. Proliferative fasciitis and myositis, otherwise similar to nodular fasciitis, are characterised by basophilic giant cells with one or two prominent nucleoli resembling ganglion cells; differential diagnosis includes rhabdomyosarcoma, which shows a more homogeneous eosinophilic cytoplasm with occasional cross-striations, prominent atypia, mitoses, and immunoreactivity for desmin and myoglobin. *Atypical decubital fibroplasia* is an analogous histological process of immobilised, bedridden, or wheelchair-bound patients; nodules and tumours develop chiefly over bony prominences such as the sacrum, the greater trochanter or the shoulder, close to decubitus ulcers. Panniculitis, fasciitis and myositis ossificans reveal a distinct biphasic pattern with a central area indistinguishable from nodular fasciitis, rimmed by a broad zone of ossification; differential diagnosis includes extraskeletal osteosarcoma, which shows an irregular lesion with prominent atypia, numerous mitoses, and ossification prominent in the centre of the lesion. *Fibro-osseous pseudotumour* of the digits is a similar process in young, predominantly female, adults, where the zoning phenomenon is less prominent. Similarly, *calcifying aponeurotic fibroma* seems to be a calcifying stage of lesions otherwise similar to late stages of nodular fasciitis. These lesions characteristically affect the hands and feet of young adults and frequently recur after excision, and histology shows multiple, more central foci of "geographical" calcification and cartilage formation. Analogous to the relationship of cellular neurothekeoma and dermatofibroma in the reticular dermis, *fibrous hamartoma of infancy* (Fig. 7) and *plexiform fibrohistiocytic tumour* seem, in our experience [14], to be plexiform variants of a fibrosing panniculitis. Fibrous hamartoma of infancy commonly affects infants, boys twice as often as girls, in the first 2 years of life with an ill-defined subcutaneous nodule and tumour in the axillary fold or groin. Histology reveals a plexiform pattern of fascicles of fibrocytes with variable fibroplasia, interspersed by loose whorls of fibrocytes with mucin and occasional giant cells dissecting the pre-existing fatty tissue. Plexiform fibrohistiocytic tumour is a similar process of young female adults and presents predominantly with subcutaneous nodules and

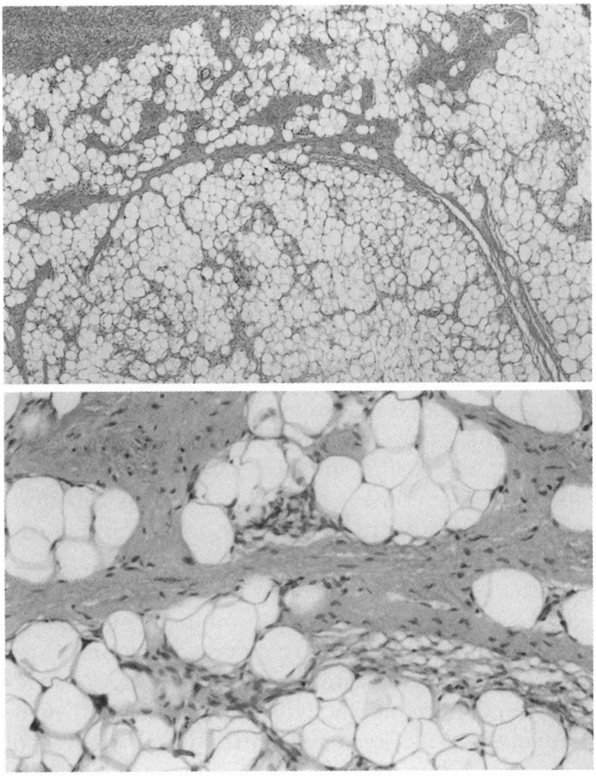

a

b

Fig. 7 a, b. Fibrous hamartoma of infancy: **a** Ill-defined plexiform lesion at the border dermis-to-subcutis (**b**) with small nodules of fibroblasts beside streaks of fibrocollagenous tissue dissecting the subcutis

tumours on the shoulder or upper arm. Histology again shows a subcutaneous plexiform fibrohistiocytic lesion with fascicles of fibrocytes and variable desmoplasia interspersed by whorled nodules of epithelioid histiocytes with osteoclast-like giant cells. Differential diagnosis includes plexiform pigmented spindle cell naevus, which is more nested, in particular at the junctional zone, contains remnants of melanin, and is S100 protein positive.

2.5 Superficial Fibromatoses

Superficial fibromatoses are the expression of a long-standing fibrosing inflammatory process [4]. In adulthood the stereotypical clinical presentation [6] is a hard, skin-coloured papule, plaque, nodule or tumour, most commonly on the palms, occasionally on the soles, and rarely on the penis. Over the years indurated cords between the lesions and the adjacent fingers cause dimpling of the overlying skin and finally characteristic clinical signs such as flexion contracture of the palms and fingers or deviation of the erected penis due to shrinkage of the fibrosing process. *Dupuytren's contracture* – palmar fibromatosis is another misnomer, as lesions may also affect the fingers and dorsal aspects of the hands – most commonly affects older men, i. e. 1% – 2% of the general population; 20% of men older than 65 years are afflicted, with a male-to-female ratio of 4 to 1. The right hand is more frequently involved than the left, probably indicating some traumatic relationship, with predilection for the ulnar side, which leads to contracture of the fourth and/or fifth finger. Yet the process may be multifocal, affecting both hands (>50%), the feet (5%–20%), with nodules in the middle and medial portion of the soles of the feet, or the penis (2%–4%), with a nodule in the dorsal or lateral shaft. These disorders are known as *Ledderhose's* and *Peyronie's disease* – plantar and penile fibromatosis are also inadequate terms – and may affect one or the other of these locations alone. Similar processes occur in children on the gingiva (*gingival fibromatoses*) and the neck (*fibromatosis colli*), other areas prone to injury.

Histologically (Fig. 8), early lesions show granulation tissue similar to that of early nodular fasciitis with spindle-shaped to stellate fibrocytes, prominent mucin and vascularity, as well as a sprinkling of lymphocytes in a moderately well circumscribed lesion; in fully developed lesions fascicles and nodules of fibrocytes with increasing fibroplasia become prominent, while mucin, vascularity, and lymphocytes become scant to absent; late lesions are similar to fully developed lesions, but with thicker collagen bundles, fewer plump fibrocytes and no mucin. Differential diagnosis includes fibrosarcomas, which are rare in the extremities and reveal herringbone-like fascicles with dense cellularity, necroses, atypia and mitoses.

a

b

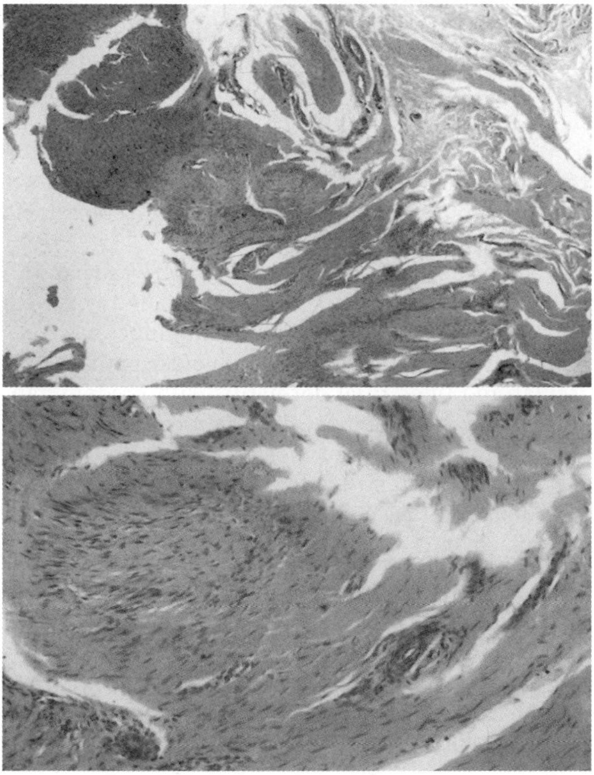

Fig. 8 a, b. Dupuytren's contracture: **a** Ill-defined fibrocollagenous lesion (**b**) with variable cellularity of fibroblasts in fibrotic stroma

Superficial fibromatoses of infancy or childhood may reveal some peculiarities rarely seen in adults. Thus lesions are frequently multiple, may affect the skeleton and internal organs such as lung, heart, and gastrointestinal tract, and wax and wane. According to their clinicopathological presentation, various subtypes have been described: *infantile digital fibromatosis* affects fingers and toes of children in their first year of life; the lateral and dorsal aspects of the distal or middle phalangeal joints of the third to fifth finger are most frequently affected, girls more frequently than boys, and lesions are frequently recurrent and/or multiple; histology shows characteristic inclusion bodies of intracytoplasmic actin-like material. *Juvenile hyaline fibromatosis* is a rare disease with some resemblance to infantile myofibromatosis; however, lesions usually do not present before the age of 2–5 years, are typically multiple, and histologically show a prominence of fibrosclerosis; juvenile hyaline fibromatosis may be an advanced stage of other types of fibromatosis.

2.6 Xanthogranuloma

Clinically, xanthogranulomas[1] [3] present with a wide variety of clinical settings: Lesions may be solitary or multiple, the latter more commonly seen in children under the age of 3 years with a predilection for the upper part of the body, including the face. The face is not particularly affected in adults. Individual lesions present as macules, papules, plaques, nodules and tumours. While multiple lesions of juvenile xanthogranulomas usually regress within weeks to months, no such tendency is observed in adult xanthogranulomas. Differential diagnosis includes urticaria pigmentosa, which shows reddish-brown papules with a positive Darier's sign, i.e. urtication of a lesion owing to its being rubbed; Spitz naevus tends to be a solitary pink or orange, not yellow, papule; Langerhans' cell histiocytosis shows more purpuric, scaly and crusted papules, frequently mimicking seborrhoeic dermatitis or diaper dermatitis.

Histologically (Fig. 9), early lesions show a moderately dense perivascular and interstitial infiltrate of slightly vacuolated histiocytes, few of which, if any, have a xanthomatised ("foamy") cytoplasm and none of which are multinucleate. Very subtle lesions corresponding clinically to macules and tiny follicular papules present with a superficial perivascular and interstitial dermatitis with predominant histiocytes, sometimes in a perifollicular arrangement. The characteristic papules show a nodular to diffuse dermatitis, with sheets of mostly oval and monomorphous histiocytes, occasionally mild atypia and sometimes numerous mitoses; fully developed lesions reveal a dense diffuse infiltrate of histiocytes, many of which show a xanthomatised cytoplasm and several to numerous giant cells of the

---

[1] Basically, xanthogranulomas are lesions of histiocytic differentiation which may, in due course, show some fibrocytic differentiation with fibrosclerosis. In this sense, xanthogranulomas were incorporated in this monograph as they had been incorporated in all previous classifications of fibrohistiocytic lesions. Similar fibrocytic differentiation in primarily histiocytic disorders may occur in the course of xanthomas (briefly mentioned in the differential diagnosis of xanthogranulomas) and many other histiocytic disorders such as lipid storage disease, tuberculosis, trauma, and foreign body reactions.

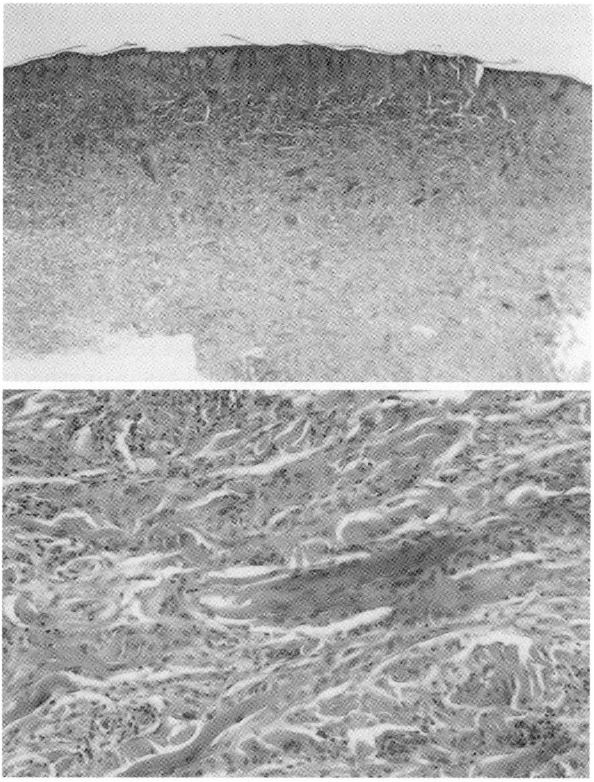
a
b

Fig. 9 a, b. Spindle cell xanthogranuloma: **a** Ill-defined lesion in upper dermis (**b**) with mostly spindle-shaped histiocytes, some foamy histiocytes with occasional Touton giant cells and coarse collagen bundles

Touton type, i.e. a two-tone appearance with a homogeneous amphophilic centre separated from a xanthomatised periphery by a wreath of nuclei. The epidermis above the lesion is frequently thinned; rete ridges peripheral to the infiltrate are sometimes hyperplastic. A variable number of lymphocytes, plasma cells, eosinophils, and sometimes neutrophils may be distributed throughout the infiltrate of histiocytes, with lymphocytes and plasma cells predominantly around the venules; late lesions show fibroplasia within a dense diffuse infiltrate of histiocytes with a patchy mixed-cell infiltrate of lymphocytes, plasma cells and eosinophils. Differential diagnosis includes dermatofibroma, which usually shows epidermal, melanocytic, and folliculosebaceous hyperplasia, frequently siderophages, and greater prominence of fibroplasia; Langerhans' cell histiocytosis shows characteristic histiocytes with reniform nuclei; the stroma is oedematous and the process frequently abuts the epidermis with spongiosis, serum seas, parakeratosis and crusts.

According to the age of the patient, the type and number of lesions, and the histopathological presentation, a wide variety of entities published under various designations fall into the category of xanthogranulomas [15]: Early lesions composed mostly of slightly vacuolated histiocytes have, when singular, been termed *mononuclear variant of xanthogranuloma*, identical lesions confined to the head-neck area are known as *benign cephalic histiocytosis*, and myriad widespread, generalised lesions as *generalised eruptive histiocytoma*. All these lesions may be confused with other histiocytic disorders including urticaria pigmentosa, storage disorders such as Niemann-Pick disease, or leukaemic infiltrates such as in (myelo-) monocytic leukaemia. Lesions dominated by scalloped cells are, when singular, known as *scalloped cell xanthogranulomas* [16], or, when generalised, preferentially occur around the eyes, the neck, axilla and groins of adult men in early lesions of *xanthoma disseminatum*; a confluence of lesions may be disfiguring ("facies leonina"). When oncocytic histiocytes, i.e. a distinctive amphophilic, slightly granular cytoplasm, darker in the centre than at the periphery, associated with similarly characteristic giant cells ("ground-glass appearance") prevail, solitary lesions are known as *reticulohistiocytic granuloma or reticulohistiocytoma*, a generalised process termed *multicentric reticulohistiocytosis*; this is seen mostly in middle-aged women and shows a predilection for disfiguring the extensor aspects of the hands, forearms, face, scalp, and ears by papules and nodules, with additional mutilating arthritis of the distal interphalangeal joints. When lesions age, xanthomatised histiocytes may become prominent, as in some variants of xanthoma disseminatum; while *papular xanthoma*, either localised or generalised, is another similarly rare entity, *xanthelasmas* are the most common variant of all types; the absence of extracellular lipid differentiates xanthomatised xanthogranulomas from those types of xanthomas associated with the various forms of hyperlipidemia, such as eruptive, tuberous, plane and tendinous xanthomas. Finally, in a very late stage xanthogranulomas may show spindle cell prominence with some stromal fibrosclerosis. When solitary, the respective lesion is a *spindle cell xanthogranuloma*, when multiple, with myriad superficial and deep papules, nodules, and tumours that are frequently disfiguring ("facies leonina"), it is *progressive nodular histiocytosis*. Like multiple adult xanthogranulomas, all those rare generalised variants of different cell types may show internal involvement, e.g. of mucous membranes, eyes, bones, joints, liver, lungs, heart, testes; moreover, association with internal disease, i.e. autoimmune disorders such as lupus erythematosus, dermatomyositis or Hashimoto's thyroiditis, or various neoplasias is not uncommon.

3 Hyperplasias

3.1 Prurigo Nodularis

Prurigo nodularis [3] results from persistent rubbing of the skin over a long time. This process occurs mostly in pruritic skin that is grossly normal at the beginning, but it may also be superimposed upon other pruritic conditions such as lichen planus, allergic contact dermatitis or mycosis fungoides, to mention but a few examples. Persistent rubbing back and forth over the skin causes everything below to become thickened. Clinically, this results in papules, plaques, nodules and tumours of thickened skin that are characterised by accentuation of the normal skin markings, hyperpigmentation, and sometimes scaling. According to the clinical stage, one speaks of prurigo simplex acuta or subacuta or nodular prurigo. When lesions are more scratched than rubbed, the surface becomes eroded to

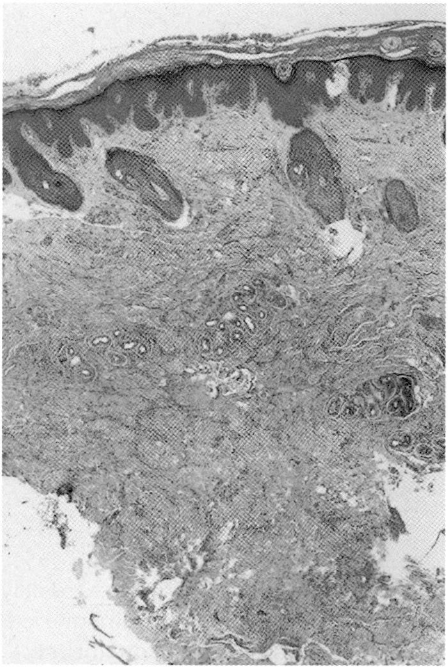

Fig. 10. Prurigo nodularis: Seemingly acral skin with a thick compact stratum corneum on the nonacral site. Note hair follicles!

ulcerated, and such lesions are known as "*picker's nodule*". Histology (Fig. 10) in all cases reveals the features of *lichen simplex chronicus*, which vary according to the intensity of the rubbing process. Mild to moderate rubbing reveals a psoriasiform epidermal and adnexal hyperplasia with rete ridges, acrosyringia and follicular infundibula of unequal lengths and breadths. Characteristically, one sees compact orthokeratosis with focal parakeratosis and sometimes scale crusts, hypergranulosis, and plugging of the ostia of follicular infundibula and eccrine ducts by cornified cells. In early lesions these epidermal changes may be the only significant pathology that forms an important clue to the correct diagnosis of this circumstance: acral skin on the nonacral side, easily recognised by hair follicles, is a clue to lichen simplex chronicus. When the rubbing persists the papillary dermis, too, becomes thickened by coarse collagen fibres in vertical streaks, i.e. lamellae parallel to the rete ridges and perpendicular to the skin surface, as well as dilated vessels with plump endothelial cells and slightly thickened walls in a similar parallel pattern. Fibroblasts become stellate to multinucleated, and there is a superficial perivascular infiltrate of lymphocytes, histiocytes, melanophages and occasional plasma cells. All this causes thickening of the papillary dermis, whose vascular plexus is further away from the epidermis than usual. Even more vigorous rubbing will also cause involvement of the reticular dermis, which becomes thickened due to an increase of collagen fibres, which are slightly loosened by an increased number of fibroblasts and mucin. This process becomes most prominent around adnexal structures, in which the individual tubules and glands, usually in close proximity, are separated from one another by vast amounts of mucin and an increased number of fibroblasts.

3.2 Knuckle Pads

Knuckle pads [6], which are often said to be closely related to palmar fibromatosis, are another version of a hyperplastic process [4], caused by occupational trauma on the hands of manual workers such as farmers, sailors, or workmen, or by self-manipulation. Clinically, these lesions characteristically affect male adults and are located above the knuckles of the metacarpophalangeal and, less prominently, the proximal and distal interphalangeal joints of the second to fifth fingers of both hands. Histology consists of bland, cellular, fibrous tissue in the dermis with overlying hyperkeratosis. Cessation or reduction of the occupational trauma will restore or at least ameliorate the clinical appearance.

4 Hamartomas

4.1 Fibroma Molle

Fibroma molle (syn. soft fibroma, acrochordon or skin tag) is an extremely common clinical presentation [4]. Lesions occur singly, in clusters, or are myriad, predominantly in the flexures of obese patients, i.e. periocular, on the neck, the axillae and in the groins, and form soft, skin-coloured to slightly brownish papules, rarely a nodule or tumour. These lesions are regularly polypoid to papillomatous, with a narrow stalk. Apart from cosmetic aspects, lesions may occasionally be traumatised and twisted and then become reddish to black and painful. Although fibroma molle may be present before puberty, most of these lesions develop thereafter. Histology (Fig. 11) reveals an exophytic lesion with a slightly hyperplastic epidermis, and at times some moderate melanocytic hyperplasia. The tight texture of the dermis is loosened up, there is an increased number of small vessels, more prominent fibroblasts and in approximately one third of lesions, in particular larger ones, a core of mature adipocytes. This mixture of cellular components indicates the hamartomatous character. Traumatised lesions may show necrosis, inflammation and haemorrhagic infarction with dilated vessels gorged with erythrocytes, and prominent erythrocyte extravasation.

Most of the fibromata mollia are acquired during life, i. e. tardive, and may occur together with *fibrofolliculomas* and *trichodiscomas*, other follicular hamartomas, in Birt-Hogg-Dube syndrome [8]. Fibrofolliculomas are vertically orientated, fibroepithelial lesions characterised by dilated infundibula from which emanate numerous cords of epithelial cells that at first are undifferentiated but, in time, become differentiated to form lobules of sebaceous cells and ducts. As a consequence of connections among the cords, a characteristic fenestrated pattern is seen. These cords are surrounded by a stroma that resembles the peri-isthmic connective tissue. Trichodiscomas are horizontally oriented lesions that also consist of what seems to be peri-isthmic connective tissue. Cords of epithelium exist but are usually not readily visible. The altered connective tissue is nearly completely surrounded by infundibulo-sebaceous units resembling paws. These fol-

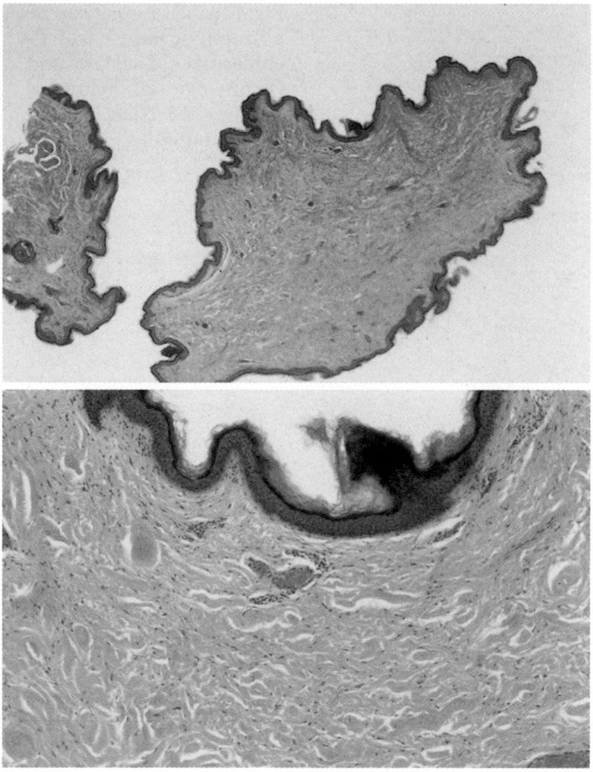

a

b

Fig. 11 a, b. Fibroma molle: **a** Characteristic exophytic skin tag (**b**) with fibrocollagenous stroma

licular hamartomas show a loosely textured, mucin-rich stroma with prominent vascularity and stellate fibroblasts in addition to the variable follicular components. In short, fibrofolliculomas and trichodiscomas consist of the same components, but in different patterns, different amounts, and in a different location within the dermis; i.e. they are variants of a single pathological process, namely follicular hamartomas. The common association of these follicular hamartomas with fibromata mollia in Birt-Hogg-Dube syndrome indicates that these lesions must be pathogenically related, fibroma molle probably being an exophytic, mostly mesenchymal variation of this follicular hamartoma.

4.2 Fibrous Papules

Fibrous papules [8] (syn. perifollicular fibroma, melanocytic angiofibroma, angiofibroma) are another very common hamartoma which preferentially occur as firm, skin-coloured, sessile papules in the face, mostly on the nose, of adults, more frequently in women than in men. Clinically, these slightly elevated to dome-shaped lesions are often thought to be an Unna naevus or a basal cell carcinoma. Histology (Fig. 12) reveals a moderately well defined dermal lesion of loosely to densely textured collagen, plump fibroblasts, sometimes multinucleate, and

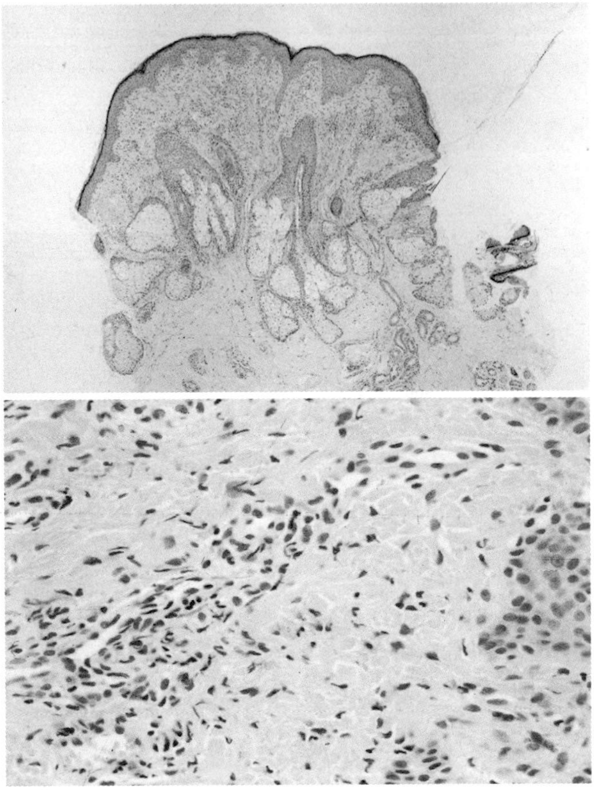

a

b

Fig. 12 a, b. Fibrous papule: **a** Exophytic papule with epidermal hyperplasia and (**b**) an angiofibromatous stroma. Note basal hyper-pigmentation!

prominent vascularity (*angiofibroma*). These interfollicular angiofibromatous components are arranged around distorted to abortive vellus hair follicles and accompanying exaggerated perifollicular sheaths (*perifollicular fibroma*). The epidermis above the lesions may be slightly hyperplastic with melanocytic hyperplasia (*melanocytic angiofibroma*). The very same lesions with even greater prominence of stromal components occur in great number in adenoma sebaceum (Pringle's disease) or tuberous sclerosis (Bourneville's disease). In these instances, similar periungual lesions with a prominence of interfollicular fibroplasia and near to complete absence of perifollicular fibroplasia are known as *Koenen tumours* or angiofibromas (Fig. 13). In the male genitalia there is another expression of this hamartomatous process in the form of so-called *pearly penile papules,* which are characteristically seen in the sulcus coronarius of the glans penis and frequently taken for condylomata acuminata. In brief, we consider the papule, irrespective of number and location, to be a hamartoma that involves epithelial (hair follicles, epidermis, and melanocytes) and/or nonepithelial (fibrocytes, interfollicular and perifollicular fibrous tissue, and blood vessels) structures.

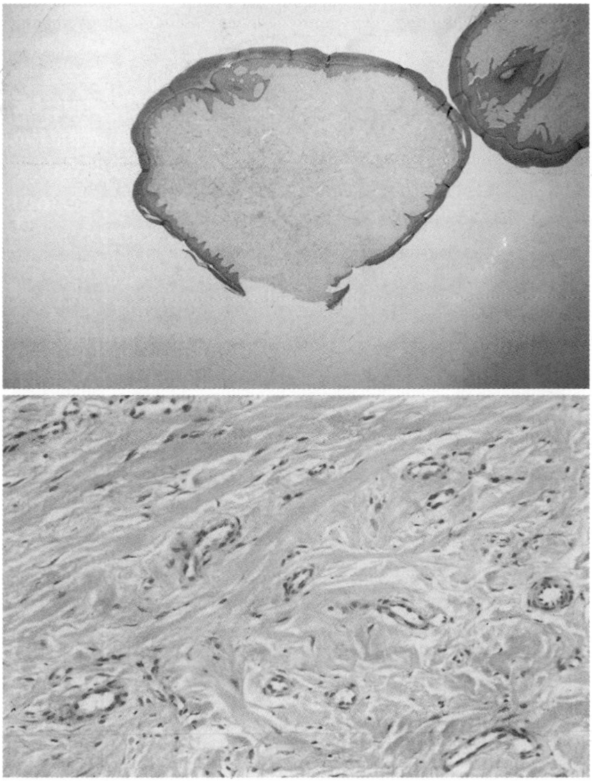

Fig. 13 a, b. Periungual angiofibroma: **a** Exophytic papule with epidermal hyperplasia, follicular remnants, and (**b**) angiofibromatous stroma

4.3 Connective-Tissue Naevi

Clinically, connective-tissue naevi [6] (syn. collagenoma, elastoma) present as skin-coloured to slightly brownish papules or plaques, nodules and tumours on the trunk, in particular the shoulders and buttocks, in a naevoid arrangement. Lesions may be solitary (*mesenchymal naevi of Lewandowsky type*) or multiple, and are then most often inherited in an autosomal dominant pattern. In 25% of patients with tuberous sclerosis (Bourneville's disease) connective tissue naevi are found in the lumbosacral region (*shagreen patch*). Histology (Fig. 14) reveals an irregular arrangement of the dermis, which is often difficult to appreciate on H&E sections. In the reticular dermis of a section of seemingly normal skin, thick bundles of collagen situated at various angles to the skin surface, including nearly vertical, are a clue to collagenoma. Another clue to distinguishing a collagenous naevus on a trunk, buttock, or proximal extremity, where they tend to be found, from what looks at first glance like normal skin of an intertriginous region, is a papillated surface. A papillated surface is abnormal for sites other than intertrigines and neck. An elastic tissue stain frequently outlines not only collagen, but also the elastic tissue whose fibres may be missing or thickened. Buschke-Ollendorff syndrome (syn. dermatofibrosis lenticularis disseminata) is a combination of cutaneous connective-tissue naevi with asymptomatic bone lesions known as osteopoikilosis. These latter lesions present as radiographic densities (on X-ray, CT, MRI) in acral and long bones which may be misinterpreted as osteoplastic metastases from prostate cancer.

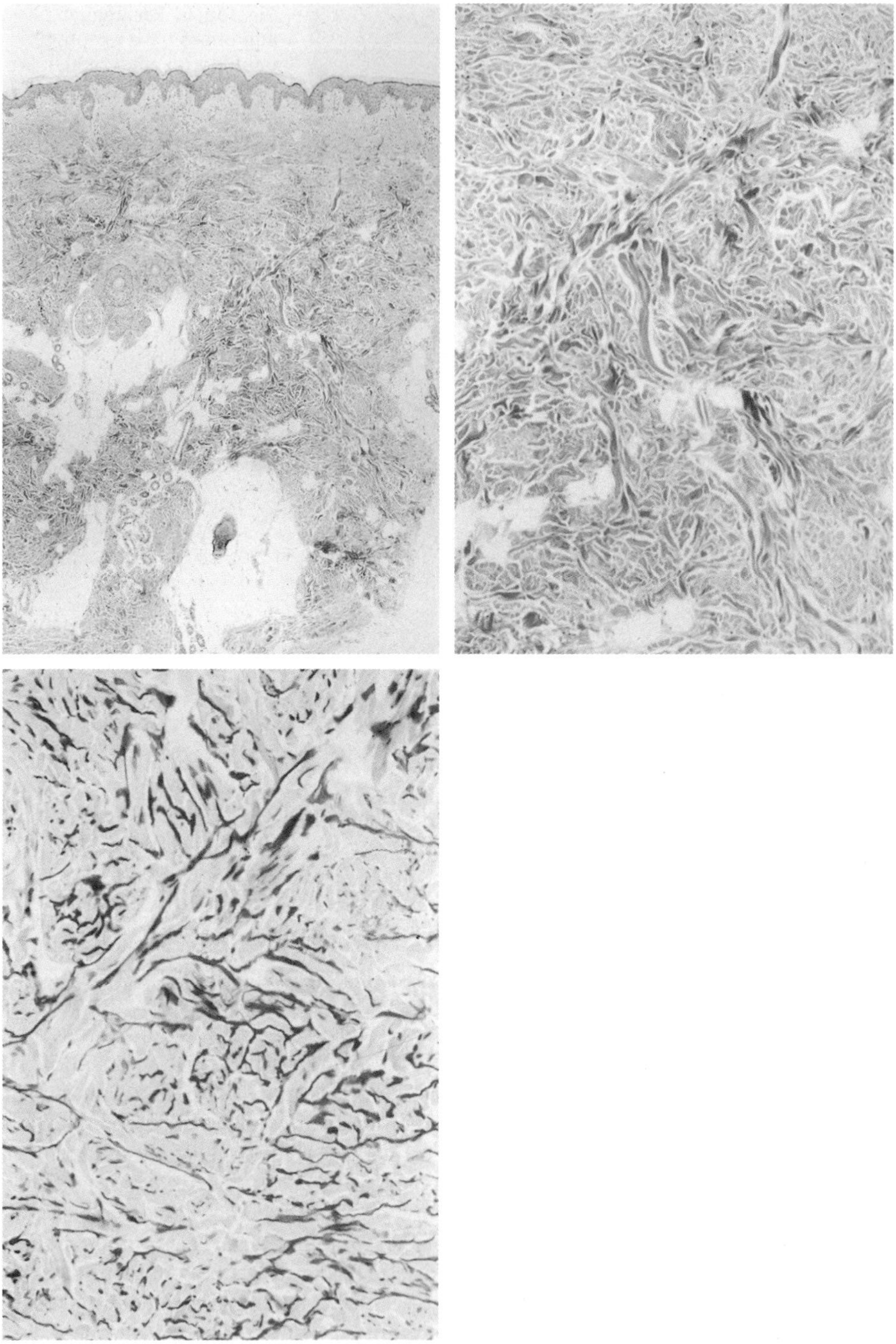

a b c

Fig. 14 a, b. Connective-tissue naevus: **a** Ill-defined dermal plaque with deep subcutaneous extension. **b** Prominence of vertically oriented collagen bundles. **c** Elastic stain reveals thickened elastic fibres

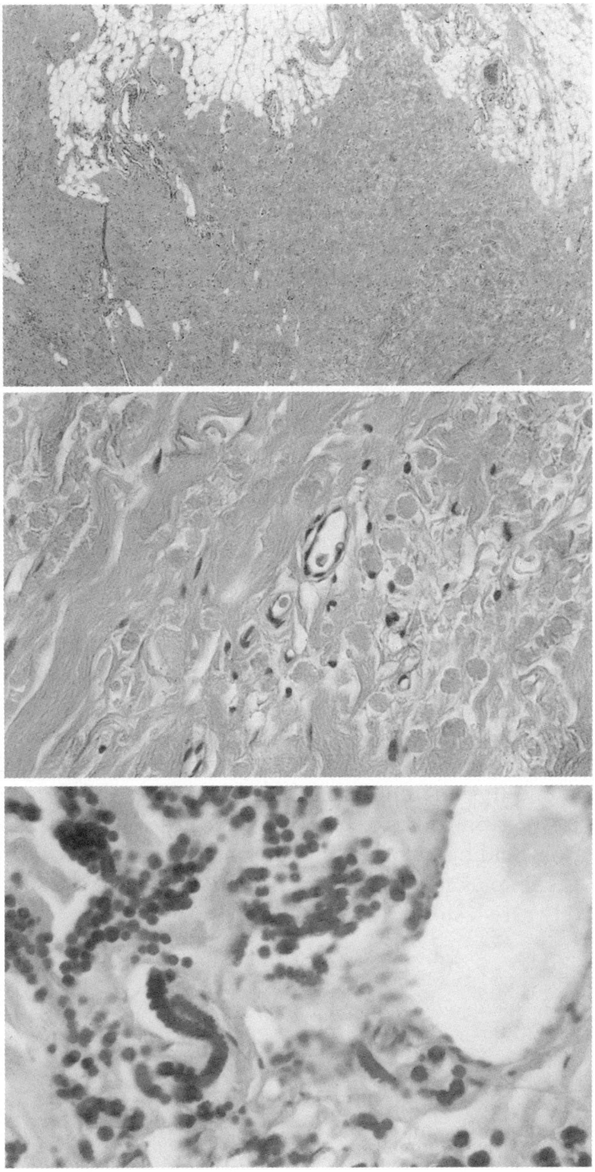

a

b

c

Fig. 15a–c. Elastofibroma: **a** Ill-defined lesion with fibrofatty tissue and large vessels. **b** Coarse collagen bundles aligned by globules of serrated elastic fibres (**c**) nicely outlined by elastic tissue stain

4.4 Elastofibroma

Elastofibroma (dorsi) [7] is a relatively uncommon lesion which presents as a slow-growing firm nodule or tumour beneath one or both (10%) of the scapulae of elderly patients, with a marked predilection for women. Rare examples have been reported elsewhere, e.g. in the hip region. Elastofibroma rarely causes tenderness, pain, or restriction of movement. There is no tendency to recur. Histology (Fig. 15) reveals an ill-defined lesion of fibrofatty components. An irregularly textured collagen with prominent mucin is intermingled with mature adipose tissue, aggregates of abnormally large vessels and prominent nerves. Most significantly, there are numerous eosinophilic elastic fibres, which, on elastic stains, are arranged as thick beaded or serrated fibres or in globoid aggregates similar to the changes seen in pseudoxanthoma elasticum. This complex mixture of components indicates the hamartomatous character of these lesions.

5 Benign Neoplasms

Fibromas are benign neoplasms with fibrocytic differentiation. The term fibroma has been uncritically used for a variety of diseases other than benign neoplasms such as fibroma durum, and sclerotic fibroma, variants of dermatofibroma, a fibrosing dermatitis, or fibroma molle, a hamartoma. In contrast to these processes, fibroma in its restricted sense as a benign neoplasm is well-circumscribed, shows clefts between the lesion and the surrounding connective tissue, and thus is frequently prone to "pop out of the skin" during surgery when these clefts are incised. In contrast to inflammatory and hamartomatous fibrohistiocytic disorders, which are very common, benign neoplasms with fibrocytic and/or fibrohistiocytic differentiation are comparatively rare lesions.

5.1 Fibroma of Tendon Sheath

Fibroma of tendon sheath [7] is a relatively common lesion presenting usually in young to middle-aged adults, mainly men, as a firm nodule on the upper extremities, mostly the fingers. In this latter location lesions may be attached to the tendon, which gave these lesions their name when they were first described. Following excision, which, due to the proximity of essential structures such as nerves and vessels, is done very cautiously and is therefore frequently incomplete, up to 20% recur, sometimes more than once. Histology (Fig. 16) reveals a well-circumscribed, lobulated fibrous lesion of bland fibro- and myofibroblasts with pale eosinophilic cytoplasm and tapering nuclei. Cells are arranged in short fascicles with a variably collagenous stroma and slit-like blood vessels. Cellularity varies considerably with areas of loose stroma similar to nodular fasciitis to dense hyalinised zones reminiscent of fibromatoses. These

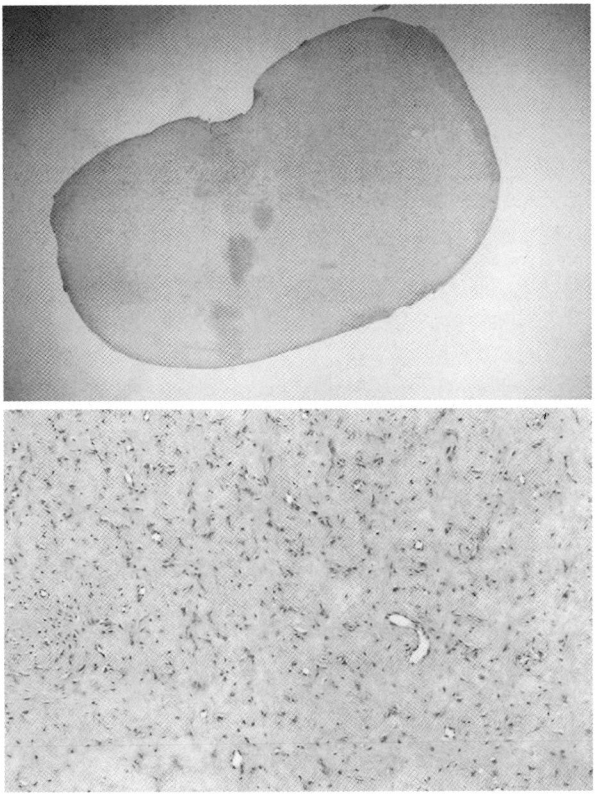

Fig. 16 a, b. Fibroma of tendon sheath: **a** Well-defined "pop-out" lesion (**b**) with bland fibroblasts in a fibrosclerotic stroma

differential diagnoses can easily be ruled out, however, by the good circumscription of fibroma of tendon sheath.

5.2 Pleomorphic Fibroma

Pleomorphic fibroma [7] is a relatively uncommon fibrous neoplasm. Clinically, it presents in an indistinct setting, frequently on the extremities of adults without sexual predilection as a dermal to subcutaneous firm papule to nodule. Histology (Fig. 17) reveals a well-circumscribed lesion with a dense, often hyalinised stroma and delicate fibro- and myofibroblasts. Characteristically bizarre floret-like giant cells are interspersed in this lesion, which is also rich in mucin.

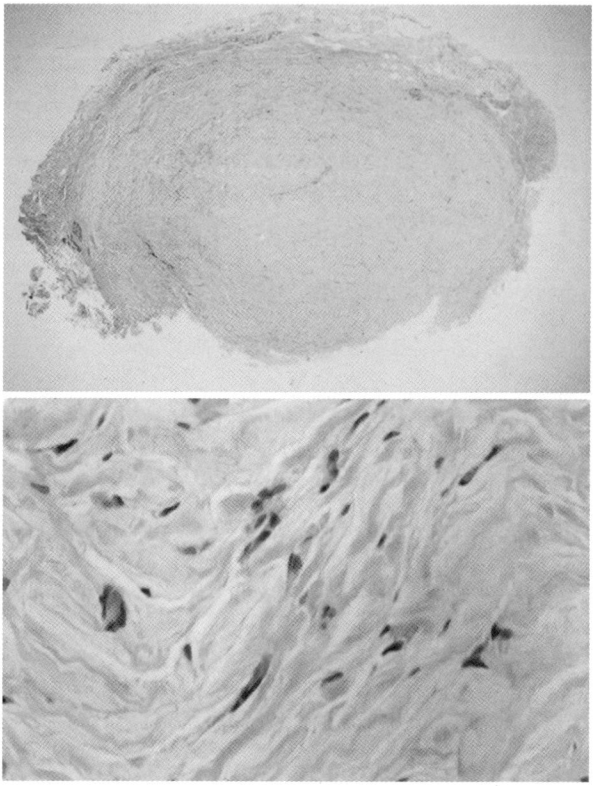

a

b

Fig. 17 a, b. Pleomorphic fibroma: **a** Well-circumscribed fibrocollagenous lesion (**b**) with characteristic floret-like giant cells

5.3 Giant Cell Tumour of Tendon Sheath

Giant cell tumour of tendon sheath [7] occurs in a clinical setting similar to that of fibroma of tendon sheath. Middle-aged adults, mainly women, show well-circumscribed firm papules to frequently multilobulated nodules and tumours on their fingers. Apart from a monomorphous sheet-like infiltrate of oval to epithelioid cells, similar to fibroma of tendon sheath, characteristic histological features (Fig. 18) include the presence of bizarre giant cells of the foreign body type; moreover, there are frequently numerous siderophages and sheets of xanthomatised histiocytes. The stroma between the monomorphous sheets of cells may be variably fibrotic to sclerotic and not infrequently shows pseudovascular clefts. In lesions with minor amounts of siderophages and lipophages differential diagnosis from fibroma of tendon sheath may be difficult; some therefore consider these two lesions variations of one neoplasm. In cell-rich, heavily pigmented lesions differential diagnosis also includes melanoma, which can easily be ruled out when attention is paid to the nodular, well-circumscribed character of the lesion, the xanthomatisation, the pseudovascular clefts, and the absence of immunoreactivity for S100 protein and other melanocytic markers.

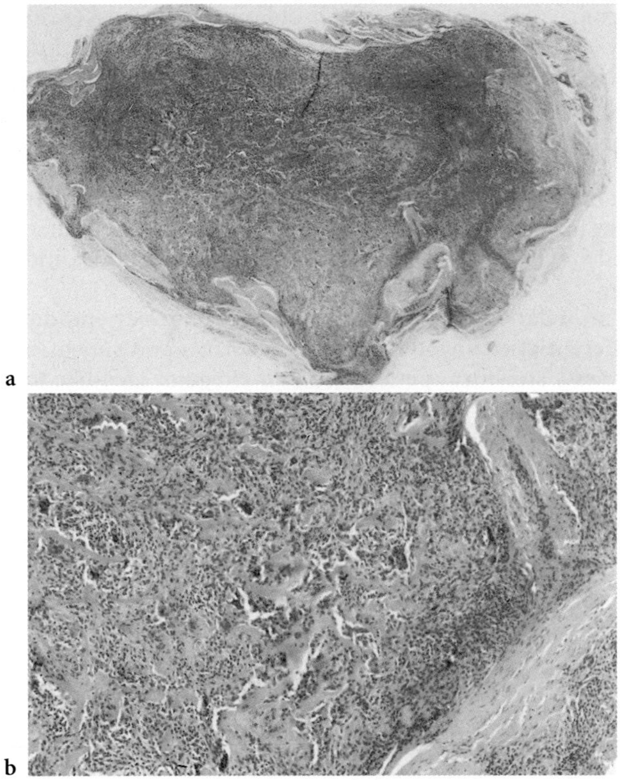

Fig. 18 a, b. Giant cell tumour of tendon sheath: **a** Well-defined multinodular lesion (**b**) with prominent giant cells and pseudovascular clefts

6 Malignant Neoplasms

Fibrosarcomas are neoplasms of fibrohistiocytic differentiation capable of killing the patient by their local destructive or metastatic potential. According to this definition, a variety of entities with quite variable biological behaviour fall into this category.

6.1 Dermatofibrosarcoma Protuberans

Dermatofibrosarcoma protuberans [7] can occur in any clinical setting but preferentially affects adults of either sex and all races on the trunk, in particular the shoulder and groin, as well as the extremities. Individual lesions may present as papules, plaques, nodules, and tumours which are irregular in silhouette and sometimes eroded or ulcerated. Dermatofibrosarcoma protuberans usually grows slowly but continuously and may be present for decades before it is excised. Differential diagnosis includes giant dermatofibromas, which are symmetric exo-endophytic nodules to tumours or flat plaques usually without erosion or ulceration; cutaneous leiomyosarcoma preferentially affects older men on the lower extremities and trunk, very similar to dermatofibrosarcoma protuberans, but lesions tend to be more fleshy and less hard than those of dermatofibrosarcoma protuberans; desmoplastic melanoma predominantly occurs in sun-exposed areas, i.e. the forehead and cheeks, of patients in their 7th to 9th decade as a skin-coloured nodule to tumour of hard consistency. When inadequately excised, i.e. with less than 3–5 cm of free margins, which is necessary in view of the frequently complex ramifying strand-like invasion, they frequently (50%) recur, in due course become more dedifferentiated and finally metastasise to regional lymph nodes and internal organs.

Histology (Fig. 19) reveals a relatively monomorphous, mononuclear spindle cell lesion of fibroblastic differentiation involving both the dermis and subcutis. The neoplasm frequently shows a storiform pattern with an irregular lace-like to multilayered infiltration of the subcutis. Cells are spindle shaped and frequently very slender, with long cytoplasmic extensions of ill-defined eosinophilic cytoplasm and little if any collagen. According to the variable clinicopathological presentation, numerous subtypes have been described: *plaque-like* or *atrophic dermatofibrosarcoma protuberans* is a flat lesion due to destruction of pre-existing dermis by the mostly horizontal growth of the neoplasm. *Pigmented dermatofibrosarcoma protuberans* or so-called *Bednar tumour* reveals dendritic melano-

a

b

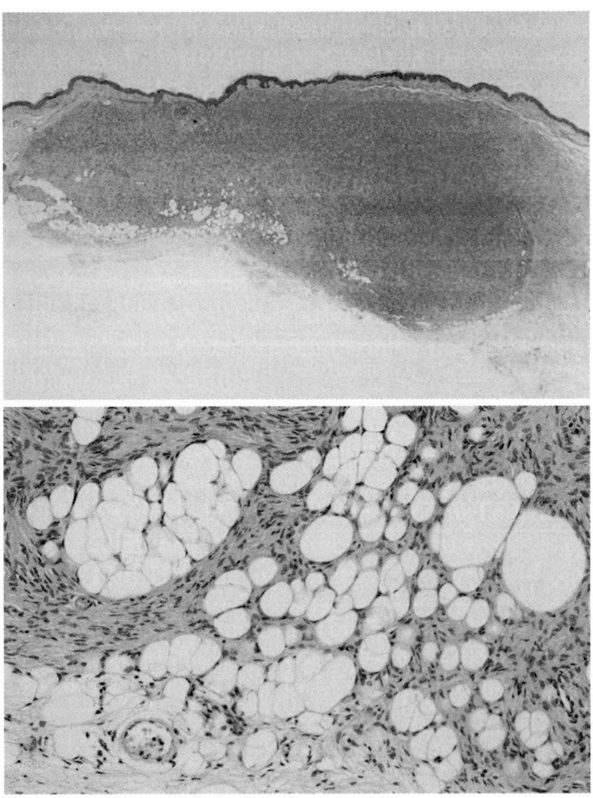

Fig. 19 a, b. Dermatofibrosarcoma protuberans: **a** Ill-defined dermal-to-subcutaneous lesion (**b**) with irregular dissection of subcutis by spindle-shaped cells

cytes interspersed within the neoplasm, *myxoid dermatofibrosarcoma protuberans* shows nodules and tumours of myxoid dedifferentiation, and *sarcomatous dermatofibrosarcoma protuberans* has herringbone-like fascicles with dense cellularity, frank atypia and numerous mitoses akin to fibrosarcoma. The latter two variants frequently recur, show deeper extension and are biologically more aggressive, with metastases and death in up to 15%–20% of patients. Dermatofibrosarcoma protuberans is positive for vimentin and CD34 and ultrastructurally similar to fibroblasts. Cytogenetic analyses have detected ring chromosomes of chromosome 17.

Differential diagnosis includes dermatofibroma, which shows a regular symmetrical lesion with granulomatous features such as siderophages and lipophages and variable epidermal, melanocytic and folliculosebaceous hyperplasia above the lesions; nodular fasciitis has a feathery, myxoid tissue-culture growth pattern, but no significant atypia or mitoses; atypical fibroxanthoma[2] is easily differentiated from dermatofibrosarcoma protuberans by its prominent cytologic pleomorphism, and myxoid liposarcoma shows fatty differentiation with lipoblasts, micropseudocysts and a characteristic chicken-wire-like vasculature; pure fibrosarcoma is mostly a deep-seated neoplasm, rarely extends to the superficial dermis and shows more prominent cellularity, much greater atypia and mitoses than dermatofibrosarcoma protuberans; and myxofibrosarcoma is a multinodular subcutaneous neoplasm of fibroblastic differentiation with prominent stromal mucin and conspicuous curvilinear vessels.

6.2 Myxofibrosarcoma (Myxoid Malignant Fibrous Histiocytoma; see footnote 2)

Clinically [7], the age range is wide, but mainly adults in their 6th to 8th decade are affected by myxofibrosarcoma. Men are affected slightly more than women. Most lesions occur on the lower extremities, mostly in the subcutis, and show a multinodular growth pattern which masks the true anatomical extent of these neoplasms. Individual lesions (Fig. 20) consist of nodules and tumours with inconspicuous, complex, ramifying strand-like extensions. Similar to dermatofibrosarcoma protuberans, lesions are frequently excised inadequately, and recurrences are therefore common, which progressively become more dedifferentiated and finally metastasise to the regional lymph nodes and lungs in 30%–50% of cases. Histology reveals a multinodular myxoid neoplasm with an irregular silhouette, characteristic thin-walled curvilinear vessels, and hyperchromatic spindle and stellate cells with poorly defined, sometimes vacuolated cytoplasm. These small, bubbly vacuoles contain hyaluronic acid-sensitive mucin and not lipid (pseudo-

[2] Atypical fibroxanthoma and malignant fibrous histiocytoma are not intermediate and malignant neoplasms of fibrohistiocytic differentiation (neoplasms of fibrocytic differentiation are the theme of Sects. 5 and 6 of this article; the only authentic malignant neoplasm of histiocytic differentiation is (myelo-)monocytic leukaemia, which rarely presents primarily in the skin as (myelo-)monocytic sarcoma or so-called chloroma), but rather unspecific reaction patterns of dedifferentiated malignant neoplasms such as all types of sarcomas, carcinomas, lymphomas, and melanoma [17, 18].

a

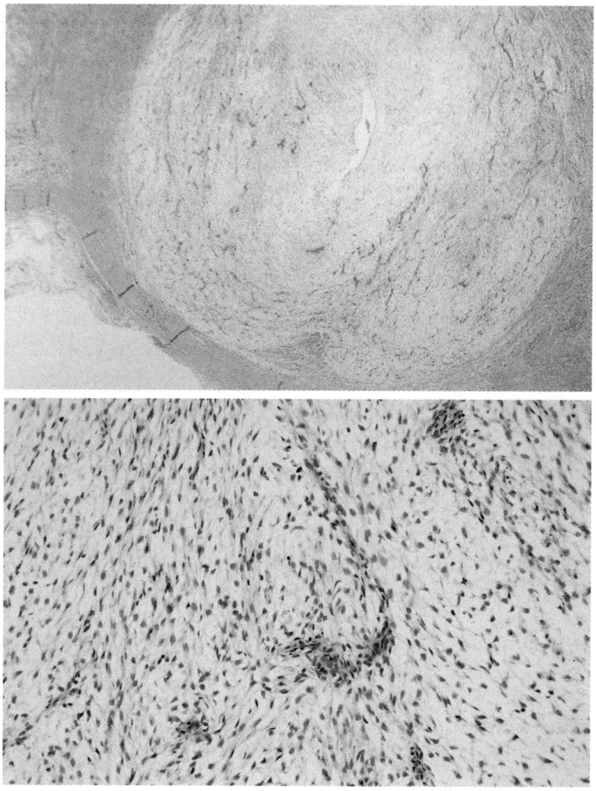

b

Fig. 20 a, b. Myxofibrosarcoma: **a** Multinodular myxoid lesion (**b**) with curvilinear vessels and hyperchromatic pleomorphic fibroblasts

lipoblasts). The cellularity and degree of atypia parallel the histological grade. In high-grade lesions, areas of the tumour are identical to the nonspecific reaction pattern of pleomorphic malignant fibrous histiocytoma (see footnote 2), and this is how the term myxoid malignant fibrous histiocytoma originated. *Juxta-articular myxoma* seems, at least in some cases, to be a (very) low-grade variant of myxofibrosarcoma. Similarly, some lesions with greater prominence of a whorled stromal fibrosis have been separated from myxofibrosarcoma and classified as *low-grade fibromyxoid sarcoma* [19]. Both frequently occur in adult men, the former in the subcutis around the knee, the latter in deep locations at or below the fascia on the extremities. Immunohistochemically, all these neoplasms are negative for markers except vimentin and focal actin, which correlates with their ultrastructural evidence of fibroblastic and myofibroblastic differentiation, respectively.

Differential diagnosis includes myxoid liposarcoma which shows fatty differentiation with lipoblasts, micropseudocysts and a characteristic chicken-wire-like vasculature; superficial angiomyxoma has no nuclear atypia but commonly shows a perivascular sprinkling of neutrophils as well as a perifollicular arrangement; myxoid variants of schwannomas and leiomyomas are recognised by more characteristic features, such as palisading or cigar-like nuclei, respectively, and show a characteristic immunoprofile, S100 protein in neural, and desmin in myogenic lesions.

6.3 Fibrosarcoma

Clinically, "classical" fibrosarcomas (as presented in the WHO classification and nearly all current textbooks) [6, 7] affect adults, male more frequently than female, in their 4th to 6th decade. Lesions are most common on the thigh and trunk and present as deep-seated and painful nodules and tumours. More than 60% of patients progress with metastases in lymph nodes and internal organs, not surviving 5 years after diagnosis. Differential diagnosis includes other deep-seated neoplasms such as various types of sarcoma and metastases from carcinomas and melanoma.

Histologically (Fig. 21), fibrosarcomas are usually deep-seated nodules or tumours with rare extensions into the dermis: lesions are well-circumscribed with a relatively monomorphous population of spindle cells with pale, poorly delineated cytoplasm and elongated tapering nuclei, arranged classically in a herringbone-like fascicular pattern. High cellularity, frank atypia and numerous mitoses are common. Some lesions may show prominent vascularity mimicking haemangiopericytoma, another nonspecific reaction pattern, or may show some focal fibrosis or sclerosis. *Inflammatory fibrosarcoma* [7] is a rare, mostly retroperitoneal variant characterised by an admixture of inflammatory cells such as lymphocytes, plasma cells, neutrophils and eosinophils. Immunoreactivity is negative except for vimen-

a

b

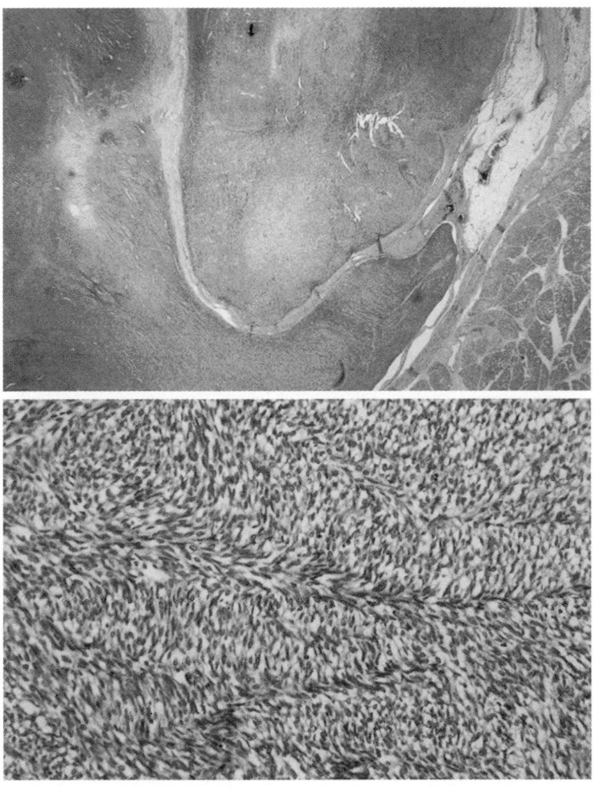

Fig. 21 a, b. Fibrosarcoma: **a** Well-defined irregular multinodular lesion (**b**) with herringbone-like fascicles of a highly cellular spindle cell neoplasm

tin and focal actin, indicating, as ultrastructural findings also do, fibroblastic and myofibroblastic differentiation.

Differential diagnosis should exclude a wide variety of other sarcomas, metastases from various carcinomas, melanoma and lymphomas by negative stains for S-100 protein, EMA, keratin, desmin, and LCA.

6.4 Deep Fibromatoses (Desmoid Fibromatoses, Desmoids)

Clinically, deep fibromatoses [7] preferentially affect young adults, women twice as commonly as men, as deep-seated nodules and tumours. According to their location, deep fibromatoses have been divided into *extra-abdominal* (60% of cases) on the limb girdles and proximal extremities in adults, or the head-neck in children; *abdominal* (25%) often postpartum in cesarean scars; and *intra-abdominal* (15%) variants. The latter intra-abdominal (mesenteric) fibromatosis may be associated with familial adenomatous polyposis or Gardner's syndrome, characterized by an APC tumour suppressor gene defect on chromosome 5q21-q22, and it occurs most often after colectomy. Most desmoids are solitary; multi-

a

b

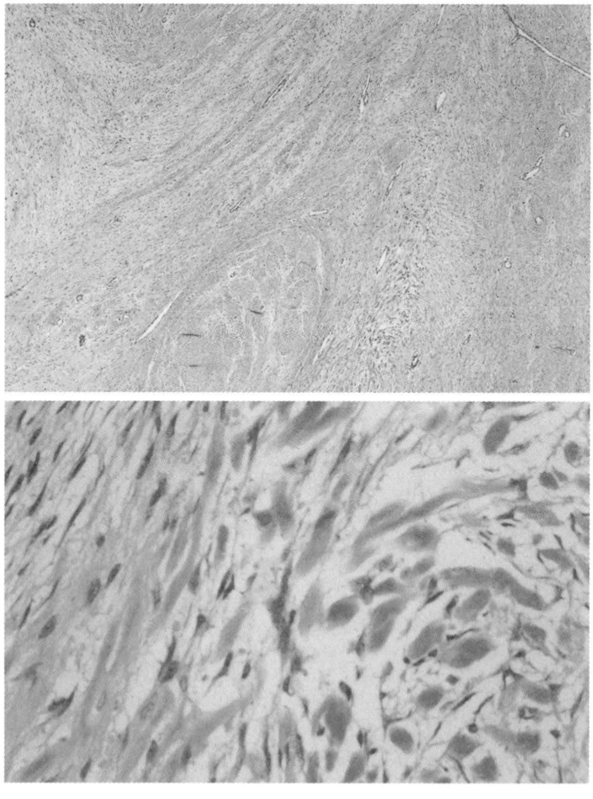

Fig. 22 a, b. Deep fibromatosis: **a** Nodules, fascicles and sheets of a fibrocollagenous lesion (**b**) with keloidal hyalinisation. Note atypical cells alongside sclerotic collagen bundles!

focality is common in Gardner's syndrome, where lesions may then occasionally occur in a deep-seated non-intra-abdominal location, rarely in other variants elsewhere. It is not uncommon for desmoids to arise at the site of a previous scar or in previously irradiated tissue. Differential diagnosis includes all other deep-seated neoplasms such as various types of sarcoma and metastases from carcinomas and melanoma.

Histology (Fig. 22) reveals well-defined lesions with an asymmetrical silhouette, a nodular to fascicular growth pattern and irregular "infiltrative" margins. Lesions are composed of palely eosinophilic fibroblasts and myofibroblasts with variably tapering or plump nuclei. Cellularity, atypia and mitotic activity vary both within and between individual tumours, as do mucin, fibrosis and sclerosis ("keloidal hyalinisation"). Desmoids are positive for vimentin and actin and show ultrastructural evidence of fibroblastic to myofibroblastic differentiation.

Differential diagnosis includes hypertrophic scars and keloids which are located in the dermis, show no infiltrative margins, are less cellular, and without atypia and mitoses. Similarly, nodular fasciitis has a regular silhouette, either round or stellate, a characteristic tissue-culture-like appearance, and no atypia and mitoses. Cellular neurofibromas and low-grade malignant peripheral nerve sheath tumours are distinguished by more consistently wavy, elongated nuclei and S100 protein reactivity.

6.5 Solitary Fibrous Tumour

Solitary fibrous tumour [7] was originally described in the pleura and peritoneum but has been seen more recently in nearly every other location, including the skin. Clinically, these neoplasms arise in adults of either sex, who present with an indistinct, slowly but continuously enlarging nodule or tumour in the subcutis, mostly of the head and neck. Differential diagnosis includes all other deep-seated subcutaneous neoplasms such as adnexal neoplasms, cysts or various soft-tissue tumours. Despite their mostly benign biological behaviour, there are reports of metastases and death in rare instances.

Histology (Fig. 23) reveals a well-defined lobulated lesion characterised by a "patternless" pattern: This term is an attempt to describe the marked variation in cellularity, the variable presence of mucin and collagen, sometimes almost with "keloidal hyalinisation" as in desmoids, and the frequent presence of a haemangiopericytoma-like vascular pattern. Lesions are composed of spindle-shaped fibroblasts and myofibroblasts with little indistinct, palely eosinophilic cytoplasm, but there are also more plump cells with round to oval nuclei, moderate atypia and mitoses. Necrosis is rare but may occur. Immunohistochemically, solitary fibrous tumour is positive for CD34 but negative for a variety of other markers, and shows ultrastructural evidence of fibroblastic to myofibroblastic differentiation.

In the authors' experience, solitary fibrous tumour belongs to a group of CD34-positive neoplasms including dermatofibrosarcoma protuberans, *giant cell fibroblastoma* and *giant cell angiofibroma*. Giant cell fibroblastoma [7] characteristi-

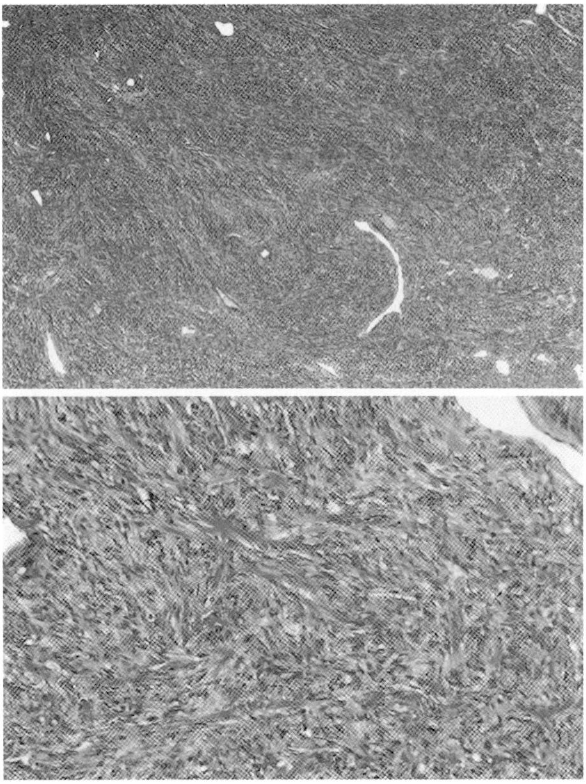

Fig. 23 a, b. Solitary fibrous tumour: a Haemangiopericytoma-like vessels in a highly cellular fibrocollagenous lesion (b) with characteristic "patternless" pattern

cally affects boys in the first decade of life with nodules to tumours on the trunk or extremities. Histology (Fig. 24) reveals an ill-defined dermal to subcutaneous neoplasm of spindle-shaped fibroblasts in a variably mucinous and collagenous stroma with prominent vascularity. Characteristically, bizarre giant cells line pseudovascular "angiectoid" clefts, and "overlap" with dermatofibrosarcoma protuberans is not rare; i.e. on the one hand, there are cases with combined features, on the other, recurrences of giant cell fibroblastoma as dermatofibrosarcoma protuberans or vice versa. Similar overlap is true for giant cell angiofibroma [20]. This entity was originally described in the orbit, since then in several other locations, and shows, like solitary fibrous tumour, a "patternless" stroma with prominent vascularity, mucin, and bizarre giant cells akin to those in giant cell fibroblastoma. In the authors' experience, all these neoplasms are variants of a low-grade fibrosarcoma.

a

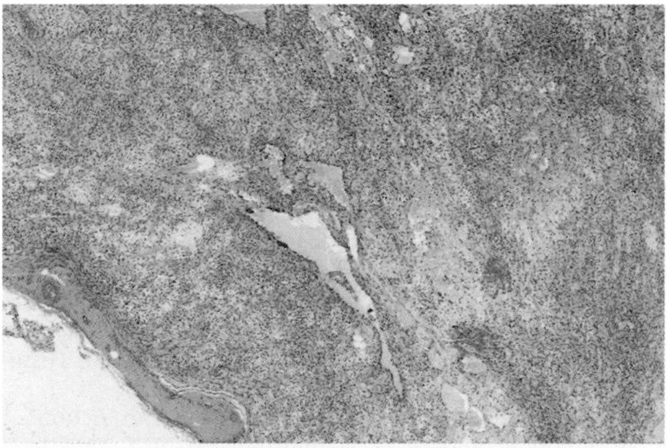

b

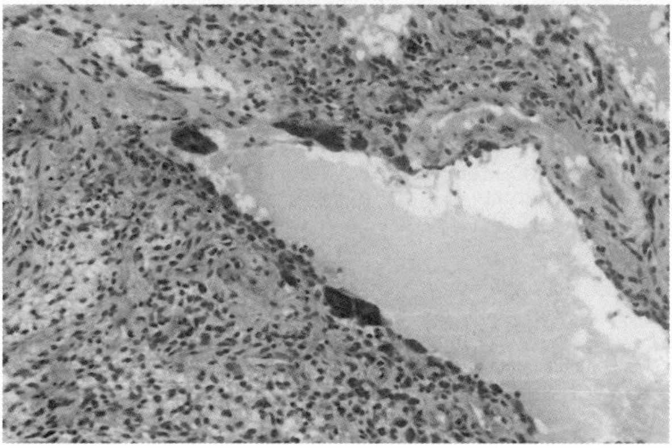

Fig. 24 a, b. Giant cell fibroblastoma: **a** Well-defined lesion with variable cellularity and myxoid stroma (**b**) forming pseudovascular clefts lined by bizarre giant cells

References

1. Stout AP (1953) Tumors of the soft tissue. In: Atlas of tumor pathology. Fasc. 5, Sect. II. Armed Forces Institute of Pathology, Washington, DC
2. Weiss SW (1994) Histological typing of soft tissue tumours. In: Sobin LH (ed) International histological classification of tumours. Fasc. 3, 2nd edn. Springer, Berlin Heidelberg New York
3. Ackerman AB, Chongchitnant N, Sanchez J, Guo Y, Bennin B, Reichel M, Randall MB (eds) (1997) Histologic diagnosis of inflammatory skin disorders. An algorithmic method based on pattern analysis, 2nd edn. Williams and Wilkins, Baltimore
4. Ackerman AB, Cavegan BM, Robinson MJ, Abad-Casintahan MFA (eds) (1995) Ackerman's resolving quandries in dermatology, pathology and dermatopathology. Promethean Medical Press, Philadelphia
5. Jacobs DS, EdwardsWD, Ye RC (1975) Metastatic atypical fibroxanthoma of the skin. Cancer 35:457–463
6. Enzinger FM, Weiss SW (1995) Soft tissue tumors, 3rd edn. Mosby, St. Louis
7. CDM Fletcher (1995) Diagnostic pathology of tumors. Churchill Livingstone, Edinburgh
8. Ackerman AB, DeViragh PA, Chongchitnant N (1993) Neoplasms with follicular differentiation. Lea & Febinger, Philadelphia
9. Calonje E, Fletcher CDM (1994) Cutaneous fibrohistiocytic tumors: an update. Adv Anatomic Pathol 1:2–15

10. Zelger BG, Zelger B (1998) Dermatofibrome. Ein klinisch-pathologisches Klassifikationsschema. Pathologe 19:412–419
11. Zelger BG, Steiner H, Kutzner H, Maier H, Zelger B (1998) Cellular "neurothekeoma": an epithelioid variant of dermatofibroma? Histopathology 32:414–422
12. Zelger BG, Calonje E, Zelger B (1999) Myxoid dermatofibroma. Histopathology 34:357–364
13. Zelger BG, Sidoroff A, Zelger B (2000) Combined dermatofibroma: co-existence of two or more variant patterns in a single lesion. Histopathology 36:529–539
14. Zelger B, Weinlich G, Steiner H, Zelger BG, Egarter-Vigl E (1997) Dermal and subcutaneous variants of plexiform fibrohistiocytic tumor. Am J Surg Pathol 21:235–241
15. Zelger B, Sidoroff A, Orchard G, Cerio R (1996) Non-Langerhans' cell histiocytoses – a new unifying concept. Am J Dermatopathol 18:490–504
16. Zelger BG, Orchard G, Rudolph P, Zelger B (1998) Scalloped cell xanthogranuloma. Histopathology 32:368–374
17. Fletcher CDM (1992) Pleomorphic malignant fibrous histiocytoma: fact or fiction? A critical reappraisal based on 159 tumors diagnosed as pleomorphic sarcoma. Am J Surg Pathol 16:213–228
18. Zelger B, Soyer HP (2000) Between Scylla and Charybdis. Mythology in dermatopathology. Dermatopathol: Pract & Concep 6: 348–355
19. Evans HL (1993) Low-grade fibromyxoid sarcoma. A report of 12 cases. Am J Surg Pathol 17:595–600
20. Dei Tos A, Seregard S, Calonje E, Chan JKC, Fletcher CDM (1995) Giant cell angiofibroma. A distinctive orbital tumor in adults. Am J Surg Pathol 19:1286–1293

Subject Index

Index of Volumes 91–93 Current Topics in Pathology

Printing (Computer to Film): Saladruck, Berlin
Binding: Stürtz AG, Würzburg